Concentrated Youth-Restoring Foods

Concentrated Youth-Restoring Foods

William H. Lee, R.Ph., Ph.D.

and

Lynn Lee, CN

Instant Improvement, Inc.

The intent of this book is solely informational and is in no way meant to be taken as nutritional or medical prescription. Please consult a health professional should the need for one be indicated.

Instant Improvement, Inc.
210 East 86th Street
New York, New York 10028

Printed in the United States of America

Library of Congress Cataloging-in-Publication-Data

Lee, William H.

Concentrated youth-restoring foods / William H. Lee and Lynn Lee.

p. cm.

Includes index.

ISBN 0-941683-10-9

1. Aging--Nutritional aspects. 2. Rejuvenation--Nutritional aspects. 3. Natural foods. 4. Antioxidants. I. Lee, Lynn, C.N. II. Title.

RA776.75.L54 1994

613.2--dc20 93-50191

CONTENTS

About the Authors

Doctor William H. Lee, R.Ph., Ph.D., is a master herbalist, a registered pharmacist, and has his doctorate in nutrition. He has written numerous books and articles for the professional health field, as well as for the general public. For example, he is the author of *The Question and Answer Book of Vitamins, Herbs and Herbal Medicine, The Medical Benefits of Mushrooms, Premenstrual Syndrome, The Vitamin Robbers,* and many more. His monthly column, "On Nutrition", appears in *American Druggist Magazine.*

Lynn Lee, CN (Certified Nutritionist), is Dr. Lee's wife and partner. She is an artist, art critic, author and lecturer. She has written and published, *Anatomy of a Cold, Dream Control,* and a number of mystery stories, as well as co-authoring books on nutrition with her husband.

PREFACE

What's the most widespread degenerative disease today in the United States of America?

Premature old age!

Is it also the most preventable disease?

Many experts think so, but the idea of prolonging life is frightening to most people because we have been inundated with the sights and sounds of geriatric medicine as practiced by most of the medical profession today.

Medicine is involved in treating insanity, debilitating diseases, broken bones, lost faculties and other horrors that make longer life seem like a nightmare.

Everybody wants to live forever but nobody wants to grow old.

Who wants a bunch of extra years if they're going to be filled with life-support systems.

We want to engage in sports, dancing, love at eighty to one hundred.

The truth is that it's not difficult to slow down aging. We don't have to rely in exotic drugs. In fact, some of the super drugs can cause more problems than they cure. (See Part Three.)

Nor do we have to rely on supertechnology or give up all of our worldly pleasures.

The natural means of reaching a vigorous 100 years are now on your table and at the local health food store or drug store. . . and you don't need a doctor's prescription to get them!

If, at this moment, you are not in the grip of a degenerative disease, the chances are you can get an extra decade of healthy living and maybe a lot more.

The Hayflick Controversy

Doctor's can be wrong.

Once upon a time there was a doctor named Leonard Hayflick and he put a roadblock in the way of life-restoring research. He did that by running a research experiment on human cells. It was complicated and simple at the same time. He put some cells in a dish, fed them food, and counted the number of times they could divide (reproduce themselves). Theoretically, by finding the number of times cells could reproduce, he could extend the figure to the whole body and find out the ultimate age a body could live to.

His conclusion was that cells could divide only a set, limited number of times. This limitation was called the *fibroblast replicative limit*. It said, according to the good doctor, that there was a *built-in mechanism that determines the end of your life*!

In other words, you could eat well, play hard, take vitamins, take good care of yourself but — when the cells stopped dividing according to a predetermined plan — you died.

And most doctors agreed with Dr. Hayflick.

After all, he is a reputable investigator and a member of the scientific community, so most scientists followed his lead and ignored life-restoring projects.

But, not all scientists were convinced. There were the mavericks who investigated further. Who dug deeper and discovered the HE-LA strain of cells named after their human donor, Henrietta Lacks, who died of cancer in 1951.

Henrietta donated some of her body cells to cancer research and they became standard cultures in laboratories all over the globe.

However, Henrietta's cells did not die after Hayflick's number of cell divisions. They lived on, becoming stronger... perhaps even immortal!

So, scientists took another look at Hayflick's theory and decided that further investigations were warranted.

Maybe the ability of the cells to reproduce themselves depends on the availability of the raw materials they need and not on a predetermined schedule? After all, if you don't feed your body the needed nutrients, the cells will gradually lose their ability to reproduce and old age will set in.

Your body is a dynamic process continually re-creating itself from the raw materials you provide it.

If you could nourish your body completely with everything it needs in the proper amounts, and shield it from the damages of the environment, you might be able to live forever!

Sounds farfetched?

Consider the following research by David W. Barnes and his colleagues at Oregon State University in Corvallis. They've put another nail in the Hayflick coffin.

Barnes suspected that something in the blood serum, some hormone or other biological product, might be the cause of the Hayflick limit. So he set about to test the concept. He developed a medium free of serum and used it to grow mouse cells from a mouse embryo.

Mouse cells usually die after no more than thirty population doublings (Hayflick limit).

In the serum-free medium they were still going on after two hundred doublings!

If the same should prove true for human cells, that is, that cells will continue to grow and divide when shielded from whatever in the serum causes the end of cell division, we could have found immortality.

Until that happy day, you have to take command of the raw material you supply to your body.

Raw material usually means the food you put on the table as well as the supplements you take.

Food is a collection of many factors including proteins, fats, carbohydrates, fiber, gum, vitamins, minerals, trace minerals, accessory nutrients, etc.

But proteins are composed of amino acids so when we think of food factors we have to break the food components down into smaller parts, some of which have not been completely identified. Therefore, we have no way of identifying the complete nutritional formula leading to immortality at this time, but the goal of a lifespan of 120 years should be within easy reach.

We have learned a great deal about supplementation in the last twenty years. We have also learned a lot about our immune system and how it protects us against disease. The addition of various natural substances to our daily diet helps the immune system maintain itself at a peak level. We have also learned how to manipulate our body's production of brain chemicals to help overcome depressive states which lower our ability to fight off invading bacteria and viruses. We have found out how to "overload" our system with nutrients that are active against cell-damaging attacks by "Free Radicals."

We have learned many things about cholesterol, and gummed-up tissues.

We have the knowledge that will enable you to live longer in good health with an unimpaired intellectual capacity, provided you wish to exercise your free will and offer your body the nutrients it needs to accomplish this.

There are many, many books about vitamins and minerals and there is no reason to duplicate all of the things that have been written. This book deals only with those nutrients which are active against aging.

Your diet depends on your choice of foods and there's a lot of good advice available, but this book will tell you about the other things your body must have for a longer life.

Note: You will find some repetitions throughout this book when certain supplements play more than one part in life extension or something important bears repeating. As a teacher I believe that reinforcing an idea makes it stick in the mind, and if it sticks in the mind, you're more likely to consider it when you're shopping for food or for supplements.

In addition, there have been times that I have had to go back to basic information in order to build into more complicated concepts. "Health nuts" will have to skim that material as merely a review of what they already know, but newcomers to nutritional well-being will find it useful to wade through.

The food and drug interaction section is a guide to drugs and diet which requires a medical discussion with your health professional before implementing.

PART I

THE WAR GOES ON

It never ends.

But, we can gain new weapons against aging. Our genes can't change but habits and lifestyles can.

And we can use the new nutritional knowledge to gain extra years and enjoy those years.

Nutrition helps the brain remain stimulated and alive with a fully functioning memory.

Helps to save your skin from over-wrinkling and can even reverse some of the ravages of the sun.

Nutrition and exercise can slow muscle loss by as much as twenty years. You can feel younger and look younger. Even your clothes will fit better and, out of your clothes, you'll look and feel sexier.

Diet and exercise, along with nutrients, can slow the decline in your heart's pumping ability by as much as ten years or longer and you will be called "The Unstoppable!"

Your bones will stay strong and flexible if you exercise and eat right with enough supplementational insurance.

Your immune system can remain powerful and ward off many of the infectious diseases which plague older citizens.

Degenerative diseases have to take a back seat when diet, nutrition, and exercise are your allies!

You don't have to passively sit back and accept aging. If you do, aging will only come more quickly. Get up and do something about it. A lot of the "what to do" is in this book but you should also keep up with all of the new research and open your mind to the truth that 100 years old should be middle-aged!

1

THE NEW THEORY OF AGING AND THE CHOLESTEROL CONNECTION

This book will present many new concepts of aging and many new nutrients to supplement your diet. Not all the theories have been proven simply because we haven't used them long enough to say positively that this concept works and this one doesn't. The same can be said for the various dietary supplements that will be suggested. There is a wealth of ongoing experimentation and some facts have been verified while others are still anecdotal.

However, we are on the road to unlocking the door to perpetual youth.

One theory ascribes all the common symptoms of aging to a gradual accumulation of cholesterol deposits in the capillaries, arteries and other important vessels that comprise our circulatory system. Another implies that it's the oxidation of cholesterol that leads to life's problems.

What Are The Generally Accepted Symptoms That Show Aging?

We all know them, perhaps too well, but it helps to list them so all of us can agree on what constitutes the aging syndrome.

- Thinning and graying hair.
- Wrinkling of the skin.
- Impairment of the hearing.
- Impairment of the eyesight.
- Tissue dehydration.
- Decrease in the softness and pliability of the skin.
- Rheumatoid arthritis.
- Decrease in nerve conductivity.

- Decrease in muscle tone.
- Lessening of breathing capacity.
- Slowing of general metabolism.
- Slowing of kidney function.
- Loss of cartilage resilience.
- Decline in sexuality.
- Age pigments present (lipofuscins).
- Hardening of the arteries.
- Heart disease.
- Stroke.

Not all symptoms strike everybody. Some of us can genetically resist some of the aging symptoms, but, on the whole, they are what we generally refer to as "old age."

Prior to the cholesterol theory of aging, there were a number of other concepts. They included the Hormone Theory, the Sexual Activity Theory of Aging, the Biological Clock Theory, The Hayflick Theory (discussed in the Preface), and the Denckla Theory.

Hormone Theory

The hormones control many of the important life functions, so, if the glands that manufacture hormones wear out, the body grows old. The remedy suggested is to replace the worn-out glands with new glands or to provide supplements of the glandular product to attempt to put new life into the old glands.

The use of glandular substances to help restore youth has many adherents. We will discuss this a great deal further on in the book.

Sexual Activity Theory

This was an attempt to compare humans and lower animals. In particular, people were compared to the Pacific salmon. The salmon swim down the rivers to the ocean. After three years, they are mature enough to swim back upstream to the area where they were born. Once there, they mate and, soon after mating, die.

However, if something prevents them from going back up the river, they can live for a much longer time. In other words, if they are prevented from spawning their lifespans are expanded.

How many 120 year old priests and nuns do you know of?

How many celibates live an extended lifetime?

Or does it just *seem to be longer*?

Biological Clock Theory

According to this theory, a complex biological clock is ticking away in each of us. The clock determines how long we are to live.

Boy! This theory does away with pollution, vitamins, minerals, diet, exercise, etc. Do whatever you want, eat what you will, don't ever exercise, smoke and drink. . . what's the difference? Your life depends on a clock!

The Denkla Theory

Dr. W. Donner Denkla, Harvard Medical School, puts the blame on the pituitary gland. He has derived a substance from the gland that he calls DECO. The letters stand for DECreasing Oxygen consumption. It is a sort of death hormone!

The amount produced by the pituitary increases with age. It interferes with the natural oxidation process within the cells by inhibiting thyroxine, the important hormone manufactured by the thyroid gland.

Since thyroxine controls the basal metabolism rate of all of the cells and tissues in the body, it regulates oxygen consumption and energy production. DECO counteracts this essential function, says Dr. Denkla, and is the cause of aging.

We say: Any Valid Theory Must Be Consistent With Every EXPERIMENTAL FACT.

The only theory that is consistent with the facts is the theory which connects *excess cholesterol with the signs of aging.*

Cholesterol

"Excess Cholesterol?" Isn't All Cholesterol Harmful?

No!

Cholesterol is so important to the body that it is manufactured in the liver. It is necessary for nerve transmission and for the production of bile which aids in the digestion of food. It is required for membrane structure and is the starting material for the synthesis of many important hormones in the body, including the sex hormones (estrogens and androgens), progesterone, cortisone and others. It is also the starting point for the preparation of vitamin D which is manufactured in the body.

Cholesterol is so essential that the human body could not survive without it. It is for that reason that, although the main production takes place in the liver, every cell in the body has the ability to manufacture its own supply!

However, because cells can make their own cholesterol, it's not necessary that any cholesterol be consumed in the diet.

Excess cholesterol in the blood increases a person's chance for developing cardiovascular disease (CVD), the leading cause of death in the United States.

Moderate to low levels of cholesterol in the blood are associated with a reduced risk for developing CVD.

It has now been well documented that eating excessive cholesterol in the diet will raise blood cholesterol and that eliminating cholesterol from the diet will reduce blood cholesterol.

Since CVD is directly related to the cholesterol blood level, then the more you have in your diet the greater your chances of having a heart attack and dying.

At the same time, your chances of suffering from this disease are lessened by eating a diet which contains no cholesterol. HOWEVER, UNLESS YOU'RE A STRICT VEGETARIAN WHO EATS NO DAIRY PRODUCTS OR EGGS, IT IS VIRTUALLY IMPOSSIBLE TO COMPLETELY ELIMINATE CHOLESTEROL FROM THE DIET!

Cholesterol is found in all dietary products of animal origin.

This includes:

- All meats and meat products.
- Fish and seafoods.
- Eggs and dairy products.
- Lard, tallow and all food products containing one or more of these ingredients.

There is no cholesterol in foods or food products whose ingredients are derived totally from plants.

Animal brains contain the highest natural concentrations of cholesterol. The most commonly consumed, next-highest sources are eggs and organ meats, such as liver.

All meats, fat or lean, including chicken, fish, turkey, and seafood contain cholesterol in fairly high amounts. Likewise, all dairy products, especially those made from the fat portion of milk, such as butter, cheese, cream, and ice cream.

If you don't think you consume cholesterol, take a look at this chart.

It shows you how many milligrams of cholesterol are in about *three ounces of solid food* or about *three ounces of liquid*.

Beef	70 milligrams of cholesterol
Pork	70
Lamb	70
Chicken (no skin)	60
Turkey (no skin)	82
Haddock	60
Halibut	50
Tuna	63
Crab	100
Shrimp	150
Lobster	200
Cheddar Cheese	27
Liver	300
Egg (one)	353
Kidney	680
Brains	1700 and higher
Milk	40
Cheese pizza	600 (12"size)
Usual size steak (8 oz.)	208
Hamburger, 6 oz.	162
Beef liver	516
Chicken liver, 6 oz.	1072

So. . . two eggs for breakfast and a cheeseburger for lunch with a glass of milk at bedtime and you've had a whopping 962 mg of cholesterol and we haven't counted any snacks.

But, If Cholesterol Is So Important, How Does It Hurt Us?

The primary cause of heart and blood vessel disease is atherosclerosis. It is a form of arteriosclerosis or "hardening of the arteries." It is a progressive accumulation of excess cholesterol in the arteries and the degeneration of the arteries.

The artery walls gradually thicken with the cholesterol plaque and the diameter of the artery narrows.

The narrowing interferes with the amount of blood that can reach the cells, tissues, heart, brain, or other organs.

Since the blood carries oxygen and nutrients to all parts of the body, if the volume of blood is reduced so is the material it carries.

Coronary heart disease is the result of a restriction of blood, nutrients and oxygen to the heart.

Angina pectoris or chest pain is a symptom of this disorder. If the blood flow is blocked completely, the result is heart attack and possibly death.

Damage to the arteries that feed the brain its nutrients and oxygen results in cerebrovascular disease or stroke. Stroke can also result from a damaged artery that ruptures.

The normal elasticity of a healthy artery allows it to expand and contract to regulate blood pressure. The artery that is atherosclerotic loses much of its ability to expand and contract. Without this internal control to regulate pressure, hypertension (high blood pressure) can result.

Blood clots are more likely to develop around fat-clogged arteries. These blood clots further restrict the flow and, if dislodged, can travel to other arteries causing severe damage.

Virtually all Americans are affected by atherosclerosis to some degree.

Some 27 million Americans suffer from hypertension.

Each year there are over 870,000 cardiovascular deaths in the U.S. About 200,000 of these deaths occur before the age of 65.

Coronary heart disease kills 550,000 Americans and cerebrovascular disease 150,000 Americans annually.

In addition to human suffering, these diseases cost the nation an estimated 50 billion dollars in sickness, lost wages and benefits.

Okay, I'm Frightened. But, I Don't Want To Be A Vegetarian.

You may not have to.

Studies have shown that dietary cholesterol has an effect on serum (blood level) cholesterol.

20 to 30% of the cholesterol circulating in the body comes from the diet.

During a ten year period ending in 1984, the National Heart, Lung and Blood Institute (NHLBI) studied what *relationship,* if any, existed *between cholesterol and the incidence of heart disease.*

This was no fly-by-night study. It involved 3,800 male subjects. The results of the study represented a quantum leap in our knowledge.

A principal finding of the study revealed:

THE RISK OF HEART ATTACK DEATHS DROPPED 2% FOR EVERY 1% REDUCTION IN SERUM CHOLESTEROL.

So, if you can reduce your serum cholesterol 1%, you increase your chances of not having a heart attack by 2%. Therefore, a 10 to 15% reduction in serum cholesterol gives you a 20 to 30% better chance at life.

THIS COULD MEAN THAT AS MANY AS 150,000 PEOPLE COULD LIVE LONGER AND MORE FRUITFUL LIVES.

AND WE COULD SAVE 150,000 LIVES EVERY YEAR SIMPLY BY REDUCING OUR DIETARY INTAKE OF CHOLESTEROL.

How Much Is Too Much?

The National Institute of Health recommends that individuals reduce cholesterol consumption to 250–300 mg per day. This range is aimed at keeping serum cholesterol under 200 mg per deciliter in adults, a level that is considered to be safe.

The panel found that the risk of heart disease begins to increase rapidly over that level.

Based on the American Heart Association diet, the NIH endorsed the following recommendations for all Americans:

- No more than 30% of calories from fat
- No more than 10% of calories from saturated fat
- Reduce cholesterol intake to 250–300 mg per day

I'm Not A Mathematician And I Don't Know Too Much About Diet—What's The Bottom Line?

You're right, it's complicated and boring.

Trying to follow that kind of a diet would represent a major change in the eating lifestyle for most people. We would have to eat half as many eggs, 20% less meat, poultry and fish and about 15% less fat and oils.

Grains, nuts, fruits and vegetables are cholesterol free, but most of us don't want to become vegetarians.

We're used to the foods we eat since most of them are good sources of nutrition and taste good and we are reluctant to remove or drastically reduce these foods from our diet.

However, rather than remove these foods from the diet, we can reduce the amounts we eat, and the same end could be accomplished by preventing the absorption of the cholesterol from the foods we eat!

You Mean We Could Almost Eat The Same As Always And Not Have To Worry About The Cholesterol?

Not quite, but almost.

You would have to reduce cholesterol-laden foods a bit, but you wouldn't have to become a vegetarian and give up all of the foods you're used to. Just cut down on the quantity.

I Don't Mind That Kind Of Compromise, Especially If It Could Be A Life Saver. How Does It Work?

Plant sterols interfere with the plasma cholesterol count. Chemically, plant sterols are cousins of cholesterol. In nature, they are found in a multitude of vegetables including grains, nuts, seeds, and fruits. There are a large number of them but the ones we are most interested in as far as cholesterol control is concerned are called beta-sitosterol, stigmasterol, and campesterol. Collectively these cholesterol-blockers are known as *phytosterols*.

Although we still are not sure exactly how they do the job, there are a number of theories.

1. They combine with dietary cholesterol to make an undigestible mass that then passes out of the body with the rest of the waste material, without being absorbed.
2. They help to make the cholesterol itself insoluble.
3. They prevent the cholesterol from being absorbed in the intestine.

Whichever, they do delay and reduce the absorption of dietary cholesterol into the bloodstream. The result is less cholesterol in the blood and a lower cholesterol count which could add decades of youthful, disease-free middle-age to your life!

What's It Called?
Where Do I Get It?
How And When Do I Take It?

Phytosterols are on the market under a number of names. Ask about them at your health food store or your pharmacy.

Make sure what you get contains all three phytosterols (beta-sitosterol, stigmasterol, campesterol).

Since the basic action of phytosterols is to interfere with dietary cholesterol, it should be taken either immediately before or with a meal. Assuming an individual eats three times a day, approximately 100 mg would be taken as a dietary supplement at each meal.

If you object to taking supplements, you can also obtain phytosterols from commonly used oils such as soybean oil, cottonseed oil, sunflower oil, sesame oil, olive oil, safflower oil, canola oil, with corn oil having the highest level. Also increase your intake of vegetables and nuts.

Get unprocessed, cold-pressed oil since the standard processing of oils removes most of the phytosterols.

The difficulty in using oil, however, is the large amounts needed to handle the cholesterol content of a meal and the number of calories found in oils compared to the use of supplements. It will help, however, to use these oils instead of oils which offer none of the benefits.

Phytosterols are just one of the nutritional weapons available to us. From fish to avocados, the world of nature is on our side.

It's a good thing because the earliest stages of hardening of the arteries can be seen in teenagers who have high cholesterol levels in their blood. *Doctors say efforts to control this lethal condition should begin during childhood.*

The Avocado–A Natural Cholesterol Fighter, As Is Garlic

If there was a label on the avocado similar to the label on a bottle of vitamins or a box of breakfast cereal, it would read like this:

Serving size – 1/2 Typical Avocado, about 3 oz.

Calories	150
Protein	2 grams
Carbohydrate	6 grams
Fat	14 grams
Saturated Fatty Acids	2 grams
Polyunsaturated Fatty Acids	2 grams
Cholesterol	0
Sodium	10 mg
Potassium	1/2 mg

PERCENTAGE U.S. RECOMMENDED DAILY ALLOWANCE

Protein	2
Vitamin A	10
Vitamin C	10
Vitamin B^1	6
Vitamin B^2	6
Niacin	8
Iron	6
Vitamin E	4
Vitamin B^6	10
Folic Acid	15

Phosphorus	4
Magnesium	8
Zinc	2
Copper	10
Pantothenic acid	8

It may come as a surprise to most people that some foods have been designed by the best nutritionist in the heavens as an answer to many of today's key nutrition problems.

The avocado provides fiber equivalent to whole wheat bread. And, 85% of its fat is unsaturated. When a group of Florida men went on an avocado-feeding test, more than half of them lost body weight and their cholesterol levels decreased significantly. Even though their diet increased in fat and calorie intake, their cholesterol levels dropped *between 9 and 43%.*

The reason I'm writing about the common avocado is because Jane E. Brody's column in *The New York Times,* March 1987, had a headline, "Cholesterol Drug Hailed As Treatment Breakthrough." It's called *lovastatin.*

Do You Know How It Works?

It disrupts the manufacture of cholesterol in the liver!

The phytosterols don't hurt the body. They only combine with cholesterol and prevent it from entering the bloodstream, so it leaves via the natural waste removal system.

Avocados don't hurt the body either. They're food, but they're able to help lower serum cholesterol.

But the drug lovastatin gets into the liver and interferes with a natural process!

What Else Does It Do? How Long Will It Take To Find Out About Any Side Effects?

According to an illustration accompanying the column, the drug blocks a vital enzyme and prevents the liver from doing the manufacturing job it was intended to do. To compensate for the need for a cholesterol supply, the liver removes the cholesterol from the bloodstream.

But, we know that cholesterol is vital to the life of the cells and tissues.

How much cholesterol should be taken out of the bloodstream and what happens to the patient if that amount is exceeded?

When it comes down to a comparison between lovastatin and an avocado, I'm going to choose the avocado.

I hope you will too!

The avocado is not the only natural food to be used as part of your cholesterol-lowering regular diet. Garlic is another.

In countries where garlic is consumed regularly and copiously, the health benefits are conspicuous.

The incidence of heart disease is very low.

Garlic demonstrably lowers total cholesterol levels.

Garlic is associated with higher HDL (High Density Lipids) which is the beneficial form of cholesterol, and lower LDL (Low Density Lipids), the dangerous form of cholesterol.

The use of garlic as a health protection food is not new. Back in 3748 B.C., ancient Egypt experienced the first sit-down strike in history. Slaves working on the great pyramid of Cheops stopped work because their ration of garlic had been cancelled. Even though they were slaves and could be put to death, their regard for the daily use of garlic was so great that death was preferable to going without it.

In countries where copious amounts of garlic are consumed on a regular basis, the incidence of heart disease is very low. Many people also believe that it protects the body against strokes, cancer, and diabetes, as well as possessing antibiotic-like qualities.

The Tagore Medical College in India selected 62 heart patients and divided them into two groups. One group consumed garlic on a regular basis. After eight months, the garlic-eaters had significant decreases in triglycerides (blood fats), cholesterol, and the threat of heart attack.

In contrast, the control group's cholesterol level showed no change!

Other researchers have found that garlic oil can inhibit clot formation, a deterrent in itself to heart attacks and strokes.

Garlic oil has repeatedly been shown to have a cholesterol-lowering activity in both healthy people and cardiac patients.

Garlic, although highly odoriferous, can also contribute to an enjoyment of the "longer life."

Roman aristocracy fueled their night-long orgies with garlic because of its power to recharge sex organs, remove sexual inhibitions and maximize pleasure in sexual activity.

The Rabbis, in ancient times, suggested eating garlic on the night of the Sabbath which was devoted to marital pleasures.

In the centuries-old Hindu books, a favorite aphrodisiac is the combined power of garlic and roses. This "magic potion" — according to the ANCIENT BOOKS — will increase sexual desire and performance, fade wrinkles, melt away bulging fat, and make a person appear years younger.

Here is how to make this "youth-restoring elixir":

Peel one entire head of garlic (the whole head not one clove).

Slightly crush the garlic and place it in a large jar.

Add raw natural honey, enough to cover.

Take two handfuls of fresh rose petals and crush them.

Place the rose petals in a pot and cover them with boiling water.

Let steep for ten minutes, covered.

Add the hot rose petal solution to the garlic-honey mixture.

Stir gently and let stand for two days.

Directions:

For wrinkles— Take three tablespoons of the elixir and dilute with three tablespoons of warm water. Smooth on face and let stand for 20 minutes. Rinse off with warm water and pat dry.

For weight loss— Take one tablespoonful immediately before eating.

To increase sexual pleasure— BOTH PARTNERS should take one tablespoonful just before beginning an amorous contact.

Is it possible that we are finally waking up to the positive effects of garlic-eating? After well over 4,000 years, the medical community is investigating the amazing concept of food for health. Scientific people are not convinced until they see clinical proof of garlic's performance in relation to specific ailments.

According to the National Institute of Health, more than 20 million adults have high blood pressure (hypertension) with almost 40% of the cases undetected.

A blood pressure reading for adults that is considered to be in the normal range is 120 over 80. Somewhat higher pressures can be considered to be normal in older people.

A better understanding of blood pressure is needed so that the seriousness of the situation can be considered.

Blood pressure can be compared to water flowing through a garden hose. The hose has a nozzle on the end which can be widened or narrowed. If it is narrow, the pressure within the hose is increased. This is the case when arteries become clogged with cholesterol deposits. However, the body is a closed system. When pressure is exerted in the circulatory canals, pressure is felt not only on the vessel walls but on the heart itself. It causes the heart to pump harder than it normally would. The arteries become less elastic and the heart may become enlarged and weakened.

High blood pressure speeds up the process of arteriosclerosis and increases the risk of stroke.

High blood pressure is just the beginning of more serious problems!

Other factors contribute to high blood pressure. It can be caused or made worse by our emotions, excitement, anger, stress, anxiety and tension. These conditions can be further complicated by the toxic effects of smoking, drinking and excess weight.

What is the world doing to solve the problem?

For one thing, as I said, investigations continue to show that garlic is a safe and proven way to help lower high blood pressure:

A. In India, a study conducted by Dr. Sainani and Dr. Desai showed that garlic and onions had a positive effect on the prevention of arteriosclerosis and consequently on high blood pressure and heart disease.

B. Dr. R.C. Jain of the University of Benghazi, found, in animal studies, that garlic can prevent plaque formation in arteries and help prevent occurrence of arteriosclerosis. In human tests, garlic reduced cholesterol blood serum content and slowed blood coagulation (when platelets do not clump together quickly, the likelihood of dangerous clots is reduced.)

C. At the University of Geneva, Dr. F.G. Piotrowski used garlic on 100 patients with abnormally high blood pressure with excellent results. The high blood pressure was lowered in 40% of his hypertensive patients. Symptoms such as dizziness, angina pains, and headaches were alleviated with the garlic therapy.

D. Professor Hans Reuter of Cologne, Germany demonstrated that garlic helped clear fat from the blood vessels of people who indulge in fatty diets. Dr. Reuter also found that garlic kills the bacteria that cause tuberculosis and diphtheria.

E. According to the *American Journal of Clinical Nutrition,* garlic discriminates between HDL (high density lipoprotein) and LDL (low density lipoprotein). HDL is the healthy cholesterol on its way to the liver for disposal. LDL is unhealthy cholesterol that can collect on arterial walls.

   It was found that garlic actually increases the percentage of HDL and reduces the percentage of LDL.

   Since it is the LDL that begins building up on the walls of your arteries, increasing the chances of arteriosclerosis, high blood pressure and heart attack, reducing the percentage works wonders in your favor.

F. In 1981, biochemist Amar Makheja, Ph.D., of the George Washington University School of Medicine in Washington D.C., studied garlic's ability to prevent clots that could lead to a heart attack. The doctor said that the ingredients in garlic — adenosine, allicin, and a sulphur compound — may block a clotting agent called thromboxane, and that may be the reason regular consumption of garlic can prevent coronary thrombosis.

G. The University of Michigan ran a study to find out if eating garlic's powerful oil in a capsule form could reduce cholesterol levels as much as if you ate the cloves of garlic. Dr. A. Tsai, Ph.D. and J. Kelley found that when laboratory animals were fed a diet that was moderately high in cholesterol but also included capsules of garlic oil, the cholesterol levels were slightly raised but still remained within normal limits.

   Other laboratory animals fed the same diet but without the garlic oil showed a 23% increase in serum cholesterol!

H. In 1975, a study done by the Wistar Institute of Anatomy and Biology showed that rabbits fed a special diet designed to cause hardening of the arteries by including large doses of cholesterol-containing foods, but with the addition of garlic oil, ended up reducing levels of cholesterol by as much as 10%.

   What was even more remarkable was that the average fatty deposit on the inner walls of the blood vessels was reduced between 15% and 45%.

I. Human volunteers participated in a test made at the Department of Pharmacology and Medicine, S.N. Medical College, Agra, India. Ten healthy people ate a high-fat meal. Cholesterol levels were measured four hours later and were dangerously high. However, when the experiment was repeated with garlic (either raw or cooked), cholesterol levels stayed within the low-normal range.

J. According to the journal *Atherosclerosis*, 29:125, 1978, the cholesterol-lowering effect of garlic has a definite relation to the amount of garlic eaten. The more garlic you eat the better the effect on serum cholesterol.

K. *The Indian Journal of Medical Research*, 69:776, 1979, compared three groups of vegetarians who consumed small amounts, large amounts and no garlic at all. The fasting cholesterol levels were 172 for the vegetarians who ate small amounts of garlic, 158 for those who ate large amounts, but 208 for the group which didn't eat any garlic at all.

The only difference in the diets was garlic and onions. Further, the blood of the group that didn't eat garlic and onions was found to be more sluggish and tended to clot more quickly.

Remember, this study was done on people who ate no meat at all.

L. According to the *Journal of Human Nutrition*, 34:2100, 1981, Bordia compared two groups of patients with coronary-artery disease over a ten month period. The group receiving garlic supplements had steadily decreasing levels of fats in the blood that were associated with heart disease. The control group, which did not get garlic in supplemental form, continued to have an elevated cholesterol level.

NOTE: Onions are garlic-related. Dr. Gurewich, director of the Vascular Laboratory at St. Elizabeth's Hospital in Boston, found that the juice of one white or yellow onion taken on a daily basis can raise HDL cholesterol (the good cholesterol) by as much as 30% in people with low HDL.

What Makes Garlic Work?

Numerous researchers have said that the active ingredient in garlic called Allicin (allyl allylthiosulfinate) is responsible for its beneficial effects. But, there is also another consideration. Garlic has a high content of the essential mineral selenium. It is a strong antioxidant that helps to stimulate the body's immunological system and helps to eliminate free radicals. But that may have more to do with its ability to fight bacteria and may account for its anticancer reputation.

It's strange that this member of the Lily family, cultivated for more than 5,000 years, used in cooking, as an antiseptic, and even to keep vampires and werewolves at a distance, may turn out to be one of the best lifesavers nature has provided.

Try minced raw garlic mixed with mashed avocado.

Chop garlic over a salad.

Minced garlic and brown rice can be a delight.

Or, mix it with a little olive oil on bread instead of butter.

For sore throats or cough, make garlic syrup by covering minced garlic on a spoon with maple syrup or honey. Chew the mixture, then swallow.

Make a garlic tea by adding a crushed clove plus the juice of half a lemon to one cup of hot water.

Garlic is magic. According to Homer's *Odyssey*, Ulysses was able to fight off the black magic of the sorceress Circe, who had turned his men into pigs, with the aid of a magic herb called "Moly." Modern botanists have named certain species of wild garlic *Allium Moly*. Circe was so taken by Ulysses' ability to resist her that she fell in love with him and set his men free.

I think we'll have to settle for just being cholesterol-free.

Even if Cholesterol Doesn't Kill You. . .

It can cause impotence in the male!

Atherosclerotic disease can be the cause of failure of the male to enjoy sexual performance. When atherosclerosis attacks the blood vessels that supply blood to the nerves that enable arousal, making love has to go by the wayside.

According to the British medical journal *Lancet,* 1:181:85, medical researcher R. Virag studied 440 men suffering from potency problems. Practically all of them had high cholesterol levels.

Your poor hearing may be caused by cholesterol and other debris clogging the arteries that supply blood to the inner ear.

This can also cause you to be dizzy and lose your balance. According to the *Archives of Otolaryngology*, 91:424:70.

Lecithin has proved to be beneficial in controlling cholesterol and triglyceride levels. (More about this soybean product later on in this book.)

Vitamin C is also important to cholesterol reduction. *Lancet* 2:907:84, writes that vitamin C is capable of establishing lower levels of serum cholesterol in patients suffering from clogged arteries.

Vitamin B^3 (niacin) is another vitamin with the same action on cholesterol. But, start with small doses and don't be frightened if you have a flush-reaction. (More about this vitamin later on.)

If you drink you will raise your cholesterol level.

According to the *Society of Paris*, 1985, studies by French researchers have discovered that long-term alcohol consumption raises the fat and cholesterol content of the blood.

Olive Oil May Be the Oil of Choice

A diet rich in monounsaturated fatty acids such as olive oil may reduce plasma cholesterol levels. This, according to Dr. Scott Grundy, M.D. of the Center for Human Nutrition, University of Texas, Dallas. Eleven patients were alternately given three different diets: a high monounsaturated-fat diet, a high-saturated-fat diet, and a low-fat diet. Each patient was on each diet for four weeks.

At the end of each period, each person was tested for total cholesterol level.

Those on the monounsaturated-fat diet (olive oil) had a total cholesterol level that was less than those found on the other two diets. . . even the low-fat diet!

It is possible that olive oil, rich in oleic acid, may be the reason for the low cholesterol level found in the inhabitants of Italy and Greece.

Margarine makers proclaim the benefits of using their product because it contains no cholesterol, however, the margarine is made from hydrogenated substances which are just as dangerous as butter!

HDL And LDL, What Really Is The Difference?

High-density lipoproteins (HDL) and low-density lipoproteins (LDL) are proteins to which cholesterol is attached in the bloodstream.

Picture them as trucks transporting cholesterol.

When your doctor gives you your cholesterol count, he includes the amount of HDL and LDL.

HDL is good for you while LDL is bad for you.

The more HDL you have the better off you are. The less LDL you have the better off you are.

When the truck with HDL approaches the artery wall, it does not unload the cholesterol. Instead it takes its cargo to the liver where it is taken apart.

The HDL truck is the garbage truck. It takes cholesterol away to be dumped.

The LDL truck is a supply truck. When it reaches the artery wall it unloads its cholesterol cargo which can then contribute to plaque formation and a narrowing of the vessel.

As long as you have more garbage trucks than supply trucks you're in good shape.

How Does Vitamin C Influence Cholesterol?

Although there will be a lot more said about vitamins, one study conducted by Stuart C. Hartz, Sc.D., Director of Epidemiology, Human Nutrition Research Center on Aging, Tufts University, is well worth the telling.

The relationship between vitamin C, HDL cholesterol, and total cholesterol was studied in 235 males and 444 females, ages ranging from 60 to 97 years.

The study showed that an *increase* in the blood level of vitamin C is associated with an *increase in HDL cholesterol*. (The good kind.)

You Mentioned Other Vitamins. How Do They Work?

In lab tests, vitamin E and selenium helped to reduce fat accumulation in blood levels.

A study done at Meharry Medical College, Nashville, Tennessee, used vitamin E and selenium with gratifying results. They theorized that a diet low in these two nutrients would permit elevated levels of LDL with a possible buildup on arterial walls.

More about cholesterol when we talk about fish oils. But, if you're not a garlic lover, here's a bit of information about it and a few easy recipes.

Although there are about 300 varieties of garlic grown around the world, two major varieties are known in the United States. They are the "early" and the "late" variety. *Early* is harvested from the end of May through June while *late* should be available about five or six weeks later.

The California *early* is sometimes called "pink" because of the skin color, but whatever variety is available locally, it will serve to help keep you healthy while it increases your mealtime pleasure.

Garlic Chicken

1 broiler-fryer chicken, about 3 pounds, cut into medium size pieces
1 tbsp. olive oil
4 tbsp. butter
3 large heads of garlic, cut in half and half again
1 large onion, finely chopped
flour
3 cups chicken stock
1/2 cup good, dry sherry
1/2 pound fresh mushrooms, chopped
1 Bell pepper, chopped
1/2 cup pitted olives, chopped
2 cloves of garlic, minced fine
2 tbsp fresh lemon juice.
Optional — bay leaf, thyme, parsley tied together in cheesecloth.

Take a large, heavy skillet, heat the oil and butter.

Brown the chicken pieces and set aside.

Brown the garlic slices in the same pan and set aside.

Sauté onions till limp.

Thinly coat each chicken piece with flour.

Arrange chicken and garlic slices in a single layer in the pan with the onions.

Add chicken stock, wine and herbs.

Simmer about thirty minutes.

While this is cooking, take a bit more butter in a saucepan and sauté the mushrooms until they start to become brown.

Remove chicken and garlic to a serving dish and keep them warm.

Remove herbs and discard.

Heat sauce until it thickens, then add Bell peppers, olives, mushrooms, garlic and lemon juice and cook for 5 minutes with constant stirring.

Pour sauce over the chicken and get ready for applause!

Fettuccine Al Pesto

1/2 pound fettucine
4 tbsp. butter
1/4 cup Parmesan cheese, grated
1/3 cup olive oil
1/4 cup pine nuts or walnuts
1 cup fresh basil leaves
2 cloves of garlic, minced

Combine garlic, basil, nuts and oil in a blender and blend until the leaves are finely chopped.

Place in a bowl and add the cheese.

Mix well.

Cook fettuccine as directed, drain well, toss lightly with the butter and sauce. Enjoy!

Okay, I Know A Little More About Cholesterol, Now What About Triglycerides?

Triglycerides are combinations of glycerol with different fatty acids. A large portion of the fatty substance in the blood is triglycerides.

Increased cholesterol and/or triglycerides leads to the formation of plaques in the arteries so triglycerides is a part of the whole problem.

As with cholesterol, your diet is extremely important. It is necessary to reduce the amount of fat from the 40% which most Americans eat, to 20% or even 10%. Then, you have to exercise for a minimum of 1/2 to 1 hour at least three times a week.

If this seems like a great sacrifice to make. . . consider that we're talking about your life!

According to Dr. H.W. Holderby, M.D., the following supplements can be used to help each condition:

For Elevated Cholesterol

1. Vitamin C— 1,000 to 3,000 milligrams daily. This helps to keep the cholesterol level lower.

2. Selenium— 200 to 300 micrograms daily.
3. Vitamin E— 400 I.U. daily and increase if there is a significant rise in the cholesterol amount.
4. Guar gum— 5 to 10 grams daily. This is 2 to 3 tablespoons with each meal.
5. Oatmeal fiber— a minimum of 6 tablespoons a day.
6. Garlic— 1 to 2 teaspoons of a descented garlic, or 1 to 2 teaspoons of garlic oil, or two garlic capsules three times a day.
7. Chromium— 200 to 300 micrograms daily.
8. GLA (Gamma Linolenic Acid)— 3 capsules daily of any good brand, 3 to 6 grams total.
9. Copper— 5 to 10 mg daily.
10. Magnesium— 300 mg daily.
11. Manganese— 5 to 10 mg daily.
12. Niacin— up to 3,000 mg. daily. (Must be in conjunction with advice from your doctor.)
13. Niacinamide— equal amounts to the niacin.
14. Lecithin— the equivalent of about a tablespoon daily (about 9 capsules of 1200 mg each or three with each meal).
15. EPA (fish oil)— 6 to 10 grams daily.

For Elevated Triglycerides

1. Chromium— 200 to 300 mcg daily.
2. Carnitine— 100 to 600 mg daily.
3. Magnesium— 300 mg once or twice a day.
4. Vitamin B^6— 50 mg daily.
5. GLA or fish oil— 6 to 10 grams daily.

These are rough guidelines which must be refined by your condition and your doctor's advice. Some of the amounts listed can be obtained from the diet while the rest can be gotten from supplements.

Although Dr. Holderby differentiates the supplemental nutrients for cholesterol and triglycerides, a combination of recommendations may be better, since they usually are found together.

It's No Fish Story

Stanford University scientists are nearly at the end of a federally funded $1.1 million study of heart disease and fish oil.

The scientists hope to provide solid information about EPA (eicosapentaenoic acid), a natural component of animal tissue that occurs at high levels in some fish.

Medical World News, 27#13:9.

Two arthritis specialists working independently of one another at different medical schools (Albany Medical College, N.Y. and at Harvard University) have both had good results with salmon oil capsules (MAX EPA) when studying their effects in patients with rheumatoid arthritis.

While receiving MAX EPA (15 to 20 capsules daily) the patients experienced both fewer painful joints and less morning stiffness, changes that did not occur when they received placebo capsules (without knowing it) instead.

None of the patients became completely symptom-free during the clinical trials, the doctors pointed out that the treatment periods were very brief (just a few weeks) and that much longer trials would be needed to determine just how active fish oils can be against arthritis.

One of the most important things to remember is that fish oil is technically a "food" rather than a drug and, in spite of having been taken by a very large number of people for many years for the reduction of cholesterol blood levels and for the prevention of hardening of the arteries, *it has never been reported to cause side effects of any kind.*

What's All This News About Fish Oil? My Grandmother Used To Give Us Cod Liver Oil Once A Week?

Grandma was right but cod liver oil is not the best source of EPA and DHA.

It all started with Eskimos and Japanese, particularly the Japanese who live in coastal villages. They have the lowest incidence of heart disease, compared to any other group, even though their high cholesterol, high-fat diet ought to make them the highest risk group.

How Do They Get Away With It?

The answer lies in the kind of fat they eat. The Eskimo diet for the most part consists of fish, seal and whale. Fat from these animals contains large amounts of "Omega-3 fatty acids," which are structurally different from the "Omega-6 fatty acids," most Westerners eat.

Westerners get most of their fatty acids from meat. Studies done on the Eskimo and Japanese and on their heavy consumption of fish suggest that the *Omega-3 fatty acids in fish are able to reduce the likelihood of getting heart disease, rheumatoid arthritis, and other inflammatory diseases.*

Scientists have discovered that if a diet contains reasonable levels of Omega-3, heart attack rates decrease, but if Omega-3 is scarce, vulnerability heightens.

One research team (G.O. Burr and M.M.J. Burr of the University of Minnesota) was one of the first to call attention to the essential importance of Omega-3 to both animals and humans, that it could be a cause of atherosclerosis, diabetes and hypertension.

W.S. Harris at the Oregon Health Sciences University found that taking 10 grams of Omega-3 per day would reduce serum triglycerides by 61% in three days.

The Nobel Prize in medicine, awarded to Dr. J.R. Vane, was the result of the study into the metabolism of Omega-3 and how it helped prevent heart problems.

Dr. Holman at the University of Minnesota administered Omega-3 to a patient on total parenteral nutrition because of dry, cracking skin, dermatitis, weeping sores, sepsis, seizures, and a general condition of weakness and lethargy. By adding to the diet one gram of Omega-3 and 6 grams of Omega-6 for two months, the patient improved so much that she was able to be discharged from the hospital. However, when they removed the Omega-3 from her diet she had a relapse.

Over the following twelve weeks, with Omega-3 once more an important part of her treatment, the patient recovered completely.

Dr. Patricia Johnson (University of Illinois) discovered that Omega-3 is transformed by the body into a cellular hormone called *PGI-3 which acts to keep blood platelets from sticking to each other and causing clots.*

According to a paper presented in the *Journal of Nutrition* by M.S. Lamptey and B.L. Walker, rats reared on an Omega-3 deficient diet suffered impaired vision and reduced learning ability.

William Connor of the Oregon Health Science University in Portland reported on monkeys reared on an Omega-3 deficient diet who suffered from blurred vision and longer response time for nerve signals from the eyes.

This finding requires some explanation.

Cell tissue, brain cells, and the vitreous humor of the eyes contain fat. Fat is used as an insulating material to keep the electrical impulses of nerves separate so they don't "short out." Fat in cell walls controls the migration of cell water molecules. So, the quality of the fat is of extreme importance. If the fat molecules are not perfectly aligned, there can be unwanted migration of undigested food particles directly into the bloodstream with bad effects upon the electrical system.

Unfortunately, the body, in its search for raw materials, will use any available fat for building cells. If Omega-6 is present it will use it even though Omega-3 yields a superior product. If hydrogenated fats or saturated fats are in excess, the body will use them. The result can be imperfect cells, sheaths around nerves, and imperfect cell membranes.

Imperfect cells lead to imperfect eyesight, among other imperfections!

Omega-3 goes beyond that. It is also able to influence the course of the immune system. Omega-3 is converted in the body into a number of short-lived cellular hormones called prostaglandins that are able to influence immune antibody production. Although some of these prostaglandins survive for only a total of five seconds in the body, their effect is highly significant.

Prostaglandin hormones are manufactured within each cell and are used by the cell to control the direction of its intracellular activities. Prostaglandins control the activity of thousands of enzymes that produce thousands of essential body products.

Eicosanoids, which are derived from fatty acids, regulate communication between cells and, consequently, inflammation and other immunological responses. Biochemists think that prostaglandins and eicosanoids synthesized from Omega-3 fatty acids are distinct from those products synthesized from Omega-6 fatty acids.

According to Dr. Lands, biochemist from the University of Illinois, the eicosanoids are really two families: the prostaglandins formed by an enzyme called cyclooxygenase; and the leukotrienes, which are made by an enzyme called lipooxygenase. He says that eicosanoids are how the cells chatter to one another. We have to understand the significance of all of their voices. What it signifies when they whisper or when they shout, and what it all means.

All of the inflammatory diseases, said Lands, are the consequences of exaggerated signals. The same way that communication between individuals can be misunderstood and blown out of proportion, so can signals between cells go awry and cause problems.

The products formed when Omega-3 is available to the body are less inflammatory than those formed when Omega-6 is used as the raw material.

Okay, I Understand That Omega-3 Fatty Acids Are Better Than The Omega-6 Fatty Acids We Get From Meats And Also From The Vegetable Oils. Where Does The Fish Get The Omega-3 From?

The most abundant source of Omega-3 oils is in the sea. The microscopic organisms called plankton make it as part of their lifestyle. Plankton is the basis of the food chain for all marine life so all sea creatures contain some Omega-3. The better sources are the fatty fish such as sardines, herring, mackerel, salmon, tuna, etc.

The names of the two oils most studied so far are EPA (eicosapentaenoic acid) and DHA (docosahexaenoic acid). EPA is relevant to heart and circulatory health while DHA is important to brain growth and development. Both substances are found in fish foods and in supplemental capsules.

Incidentally, Eskimos eat about one pound of fish every day and the Japanese in coastal areas consume about 3/4 pound a day. In contrast, the American public eats only about three pounds a year!

And some of us don't eat fish at all.

You Mentioned That EPA Prevents Clotting—What If I Cut Myself?

Only on rare occasions would the use of EPA interfere with the normal clotting procedure and that would be if a person was taking an anti-clotting medication at the same time. In such a situation the doctor would not use both products together.

EPA helps to prevent clotting of blood inside the blood vessels. You don't want clotting there. You want the blood to be less sticky and able to flow easily through the arteries and the veins. A clot in an artery or vein could cause interference with the flow of blood and if the clot happens to block the flow completely, a very serious situation could develop.

Blood clotting involves special cells called platelets. They contain a substance called thromboxane which makes them sticky and able to clot when the clot is needed.

If your diet contains too much of the wrong kind of fat, they can become too sticky and more likely to clump together. They can also become so sticky that they will adhere to the walls of the arteries. If enough of them do that, the walls become narrower and a condition known as atherosclerosis is liable to develop.

EPA helps to form a more slippery, less sticky type of platelet which contributes to a better circulation and less chance of an internal clot.

Unless you are being treated with an anticoagulant such as heparin, a slightly increased bleeding time will not be a factor. Eskimos have twice the normal bleeding time that we have.

I Was Told That Vegetable Oils Were Good For The Body.

They are, compared to animal fats. In fact, olive oil is a monounsaturated oil which is being recommended as a cholesterol-lowering agent. However, teaspoon for teaspoon, fish oil is two to five times more potent in lowering blood cholesterol than most vegetable oils.

Mother's milk contains EPA and DHA. The liver is able to make some from linolenic acid supplied by vegetable oils. DHA is found in high concentrations in the brain and the retina of the eye. It would seem wise to provide enough raw material to cover the needs of the developing fetus, so fish should be a part of every pregnant women's diet.

I Don't Want To Eat A Pound Of Fish A Day But I Would Like To Eat Some Fish. Which Are The Best?

Besides sardines, herring, mackerel, salmon and tuna, you could try pompano, butterfish or pilchard.

And, you can greatly reduce your risk of heart trouble without turning into an Eskimo.

If you eat as little as 7 to 10 ounces of fish every week you can cut the risk of heart attack by 64%.

Or, use a supplement that will give you a balanced blend of fish oils containing both EPA and DHA.

Take 2 to 6 grams of the supplement every day, according to the amount in each capsule shown on the label. But, you still have to cut down on the saturated fat in your diet. Taking a supplement and eating a lot of saturated fat doesn't make any sense.

Your body will only benefit if you substitute the fish oil for the other less nutritious oils and fats in your diet.

Another Test Involving Fish Oil Capsules.

Dr. C. Jones, London Chest Hospital, London, England has reported to the *Br. Med. Jnl.* 293:104-105, 1987, that fish oil capsules were given for 6 weeks to 16 patients with mild hypertension in a double-blind, placebo-controlled crossover study. Their beginning blood pressure was 161 over 94.5 mm of mercury.

After six weeks, the placebo group showed no change while the group treated with fish oil dropped to 151 over 92.5. This is a 10 point drop in 42 days without dangerous drugs.

Most patients found the fish oil supplements preferable to their previous antihypertensive treatment. The doctor suggests that all-natural fish oil supplementation is a viable substitute for patients with mild hypertension who are reluctant to embark on dangerous drug therapies.

More On Investigations Into Fish Oil

Clinical Research, 1987, 35:A164

Boyden, Starich, Lardino: "Dietary enrichment with Omega-3 fatty acids leads to their incorporation into the pancreatic islet and skeletal muscle phospholipid membranes."

The association between fish oil consumption and diabetes was studied by researchers at the University of Nevada in Reno.

Laboratory animals were fed their usual diet plus either fish oils (Omega-3 fatty acids) or corn oil (Omega-6 fatty acids), to a concentration of 10% of total calorie intake.

At the end of six weeks it was determined that concentrations of EPA and DHA in the muscle and pancreas cell membrane were more than three times higher after supplementation with fish oils, compared to the controls using corn oil.

These researchers conclude that fatty acids in fish oil are easily incorporated into the cell membranes and muscle of the pancreas which might *partially explain the effects of these fatty acids on the prevention or treatment of diabetes.*

Another Study Involving High Blood Pressure and Fish Oil

Atherosclerosis, 1986;62:259-265.

Singer, Berger, Luck, et al: "Long term effect of mackerel diet on blood pressure, serum lipids, and thromboxane formation in patients with mild hypertension."

This research was done at the Central Institute for Cardiovascular Research, Academy of Sciences of the German Democratic Republic.

Individuals with mild hypertension *who received no medication,* were placed on their normal diet plus two cans of mackerel for two weeks.

The two cans of mackerel provided 2.2 grams of EPA and 2.8 grams of DHA each day.

The preliminary study was followed by an eight month regimen during which the subjects supplemented their diet with three cans of mackerel three times a week or 3.3 grams of EPA and 4.2 grams of DHA each week.

Diastolic and systolic blood pressure decreased, total cholesterol, LDL cholesterol and triglyceride levels dropped, and HDL cholesterol levels increased.

The effects of fish oil on blood pressure and risk for cardiovascular disease appears to be dose related. Even moderate intakes of EPA and DHA (7.5 grams per week) lower blood pressure in people with mild hypertension. Larger doses may be necessary to sustain beneficial changes in serum lipids.

Olive Oil and HDL Cholesterol

Lancet, 1:122-124

Mensink and Katan, Department of Human Nutrition, Agricultural Division, Agricultural University, The Netherlands.

Since HDL cholesterol appears to be protective against heart disease, there is a need to identify the diet that will lower total cholesterol without lowering the HDL fraction.

The authors report that a diet rich in olive oil lowered total cholesterol without lowering the HDL fraction in a group of volunteers who consumed the olive oil diet for 36 days.

Lancet, 1:983-984

Ancel Keys, School of Public Health, University of Minnesota, Minneapolis, Minn.

Although it is commonly recommended that fat consumption be reduced to 30% of calories or less for the prevention of heart disease, the author notes that this recommendation should apply only to the populations such as those of Northern Europe and the United States where most of the fat in the diet comes from meat and dairy products.

In Mediterranean countries where the type off fat consumed is predominantly olive oil rather than animal fat, a high-fat diet is not associated with an increased risk of cardiovascular heart disease.

So, by increasing the intake of beneficial oils and reducing the intake of harmful oils, you can reverse the amount of deadly plaque you have built up in your arteries. This means a dozen or so more vigorous years.

And this is only the beginning!

2

STOP AGING

If you're still not convinced that you can stop aging and live to be 100, you should know that the average lifespan has been increasing since the 1950's. And, in the 1990's, lifespan is expected to continue to increase.

The elderly, particularly, have had a steady sustained increase in their lifespan since 1950.

Conventional theory predicts that the older a person gets, the more likely he or she is to die.

Conventional Theory May Be All Wrong!

A sixty year old, on average, could live ten more years but an eighty year old, on average, could live twenty more years.

If the Census Bureau is right, the number of people aged 85 or older will grow from 3.3 million today to 18.7 million by 2080.

That's a blink of an eye away.

People entering old age — or what has been considered to be old age — must be in better shape than their forebears to have life spans continue to increase.

In order to make 100 years, you first have to make 80 years — after that it's all downhill!

Am I making this up?

First, read *The New York Times,* Monday, November 16, 1992, for an article entitled "New Views on Lifespans Alter Forecasts on Elderly." Then, read this book.

The most widespread illness in America today is also the most preventable.

It is premature old age.

The clock never killed anyone.

You don't die of old age. What kills people is injury or disease. Old age, as we know it, is really the result of attack after attack on the body by the environment and our lifestyle and the accumulation of the damage done to us.

It's like a prizefighter who absorbs blow after blow until he is so weakened a light tap will result in a K.O.

The passage of time won't kill anyone. Science hasn't yet discovered a single disease that is the result of time. The bent posture, shaking hand, unsteady gait, and even the loss of memory cannot be credited to the passing of time. They belong in the column dedicated to the life you lead.

And they can be avoided!

Consider the proposition that your age in years and the state of your health may not match. On average, there is a decline of faculties as time passes. However, some people remain chronologically old and biologically young. As one woman said to me, "My twin sister gasped when she compared the 15 years she'd aged to the 5 years younger I looked."

Don't believe, because the usual aging pattern is what is presented to you by people who have not followed or switched to an anti-aging lifestyle, that this pattern is natural. It is unnatural and the result of the same kinds of disorders caused by the "aging" lifestyles of large numbers of people who don't know any better.

The detrimental changes we have come to expect with aging, because most people represent those changes, is a lie! The unnatural has come to be natural only because most people do not realize they have the power to control the aging factors.

Consider the way most people have been taught that blood pressure rises with aging. It's true that, in the United States, blood pressure does go up as we get older. But when we consider the Non-Western world, there are many population groups where there is little variation in pressure as people age.

Then, what about the undeniable fact that some aspects of what we have come to call aging, such as muscle tone, excess body fat, high blood pressure, atherosclerosis and a gaggle of other degenerative diseases can be reversed by a change in lifestyle that includes exercise, dietary control and supplements?

So. . . if biology and chronology can be separated, if what we have been accustomed to call aging is due to environmental insults, if some of the "inevitable" age changes are reversible, you have more control of aging than you ever thought possible!

Chromium and the Sugar Factor

Throughout the years there has been a battle between those who consider sugar to be of little concern, as far as aging and other biological procedures are concerned, and those who consider sugar to be the Devil.

It's true that sugar requires vitamins (particularly the B-complex vitamins) to be metabolized. This robs the body of these workhorse vitamins and other systems can suffer.

It's true that sugar causes cavities.

So we go to the dentist more often and take a lot of B-complex supplements.

That's not the reason to avoid sugar, although it's a good idea to use as little table sugar as possible and avoid foods that are loaded with it. The real reason is to help control aging!

It's a fact, as we get on in years we find it more difficult to burn off the table sugar we eat. This means, unless we control our intake, there will be a slow rise in our blood sugar level. This "condition" can also be described as a pre-disease.

Why call it a pre-disease?

Because it can lead to a rise in blood fats, a rise in the level of insulin and a rise in the risk of glucose intolerance.

The major cause of this pre-disease is called insulin resistance because insulin gradually loses its ability to metabolize sugar.

Is this a situation we must bow our necks to?

If I thought so, I wouldn't bother to write this book. As a matter of fact, many cases of insulin resistance can be corrected with supplements. This wasn't always known. Back in the early 1970's, Dr. Walter Merz of the U.S. Department of Agriculture declared that chromium was essential for normal insulin metabolism. Till then, most physicians thought the rise in blood sugar levels they found in their aging patients was normal.

Chromium was regarded as a toxic trace metal. Research done in the mid-fifties noted that glucose intolerance (decreased ability to remove sugar from the blood for cellular nourishment) could be corrected in rats by feeding them brewer's yeast. After a painstaking search for the active ingredient in yeast that had the beneficial effect, they discovered trivalent chromium in the form of GTF (glucose tolerance factor).

So, now the theory that insulin production declined with age had to be put to rest. It wasn't so much that the amount of insulin decreased as it was insulin resistance. When you take in sugar, you still cause insulin release, but then the insulin "forgets" the job it was intended for. Your body then has to react to the excess insulin that is beginning to damage tissues. It calls on the liver to turn the circulating insulin into a neutral fat which it stores away as body fat.

That may be one answer to your complaint that you eat so little but still are packing away fat on your behind and stomach.

But that doesn't stop you from gorging on sugar-laced foods until, eventually, the liver's ability to balance the insulin budget is overwhelmed and both blood insulin and blood triglycerides rise, and with them the possible consequence of heart disease.

What Else?

The triglycerides the liver has stored away build up body fat levels, even though you went on a low-calorie diet. Body fat levels rise above the suggested safe levels of 5 to 17 percent for men and 8 to 20 percent for women. This increases your risk of cancer and other degenerative diseases.

Eventually the excess sugar spills into your urine and then there's the danger of adult onset diabetes.

Now you understand the term pre-disease!

Back to the discovery of chromium as a essential element for normal insulin metabolism.

The RDA handbook recommends 50 to 200 mcg (micrograms) per day. However, recent research has shown that some people may need as much as 300 mcg of chromium per day. If you are an active exerciser or more than just a weekend athlete, you may need even more because exercise can have a great influence on the chromium picture. However, to increase your intake over 200 mcg daily requires careful monitoring by a physician. Self-medication, in this case, must be tempered with extreme care.

Considering non-practicing athletes, which most of us are, we find that 90 percent of Americans obtain less than 50 mcg per day from the food they eat.

It appears that chromium deficiency is widespread in America!

Not everybody is totally at risk. If your diet consists of mushrooms, natural whole grain bread and shellfish, you're probably taking in about 150 mcg of chromium daily and should be in relatively good shape to make it to 100 years or more.

At the other end of the scale is the Standard American Diet (SAD) with the possibility of only 20 mcg of chromium.

Which Brings Us to the Use of Chromium as a Supplement in the War on Aging

There is no doubt that chromium has a prophylactic and therapeutic potential for protection against insulin resistance. Studies clearly show it plays a definitive role in promoting tissue responsiveness to it.

But What Kind Of Chromium And How Much?

For most people, an intake of 150 to 200 mcg a day is adequate. Your doctor may raise the intake to 300 mcg, but on your own, keep it at the 200 level.

Your health food store will have a number of chromium supplements on the shelf. I prefer chromium picolinate. It is a combination of chromium and picolinic acid, an amino acid metabolite found naturally in the liver and kidney that has been shown to be a good carrier of chromium around the body. It is five times better absorbed and retained than other forms. Chromium picolinate is patented by the U.S. Department of Agriculture which has licensed it for commercial distribution. You'll have little trouble finding it on the shelf.

Supplementation alone is not going to do the trick all by itself, we're going to delve into other ways to live to be 100. However, in a controlled study using chromium picolinate, 200 mcg daily, blood sugar did drop 18% after only six weeks.

(Evans, G.W., "The effects of chromium picolinate on insulin-controlled parameters in humans," *Int. J. BIosocial Res.*, Vol. 11(2);163-180, 1989.)

The Low-fat Diet—Linoleic and Linolenic Acids

But you can't go on eating the SAD diet that got you into this state; you will have to switch to a high carbohydrate, low-fat diet for the best effects.

What Is Low-fat? All The Vegetable Oil You Want Because It's Not Animal In Origin?

We're about to burst your bubble. We have been told that no more than 25 percent of our total caloric intake should be fats (oil) and of the 25%, no more than 10 percent should be saturated fat. Hold that thought for the next few pages.

The human body cannot get along without a certain amount of fat, or more correctly, fatty acids. They are a major component of cell membranes and have special roles in the brain, eyes, adrenal glands, sex organs, and so on. In fact, an inadequate supply of these fatty acids can lead to premature aging. (See also previous chapter.)

All food fats can be used for energy, but only certain fats can be used for the other essential roles that fats play in the body.

All food fats are made up of a fat part and an acid part. Hence the name fatty acid. There are saturated fats and unsaturated fats. Chemically they can be compared to a chain with carbon as the links on the chain. A fatty acid can be a short chain with only 4 carbon links or a larger chain having 20 to 24 carbon links, like most of the fatty acids in your brain, or even longer.

Saturated fats have a hydrogen atom attached to all of the carbon links. There's no room to attach anything else.

Unsaturated fats have a number of links that are free of hydrogen atoms.

Get the picture?

Unsaturated fats are more biologically active.

Saturated fats can only be burned for energy or stored away on your rear end!

There are two unsaturated fats that are essential to longevity. You can't manufacture them in your body, but must get them from your diet. They're called linoleic and linolenic acids.

Here's the kicker. . .

As we get older, we can't utilize these fatty acids in the same manner we used to, but as stated in the previous chapter, there are two oils found in fish (EPA and DHA) which easily take up the slack.

Eat salmon, tuna, sardines, mackerel, trout. Or take a supplement of fish oil — two capsules three times a day with meals — available at any health food store. If you're over 55, also take a supplement of gamma-linolenic acid morning and night (from your health food store) to insure complete conversion of these fatty acids into the chemicals your body needs to make 100 years of age.

Now, back to the thought you were holding about how much oil there should be in your diet.

15 percent of total daily caloric intake is sufficient.

On average, this is the figure for fat intake from the countries with the lowest incidence of degenerative diseases, such as Japan.

There are, however, a number of classes of fats, so try this breakdown for longevity:

- 3% saturated fat
- 4% monounsaturated fat
- 8% fat containing linolenic and linoleic acid

How Does That Compute If You're Eating 2,500 Calories Daily?

- 375 calories or 42 grams of fat

In Ordinary English?

A daily total from food and cooking:

- 3 tablespoons of olive oil
- 2 tablespoons of flaxseed oil or its equivalent
- A couple of pats of butter on your wholewheat toast

BUTTER? Not Margarine?

No way. Margarine is oil that has been processed so that the body can no longer use it.

Natural oils are in what is called a CIS formation. That is, the hydrogen atoms hang on the carbon links in the same manner; all are either hanging down or standing up. The body recognizes that formation and is able to use the oil for its needs.

When a naturally liquid oil is processed to become a solid (like margarine), the hydrogen atoms become haphazard, some up, some down. This is now called a TRANS formation. TRANS molecules are rarely found in nature so the body has never had to develop the mechanism to turn the TRANS oil into useful material.

All nutritionally-important oils are in the CIS formation. And, if the manufacturer decides to play tricks and puts "partially hydrogenated" on the label, it doesn't help. Partially hydrogenated is like a little pregnant.

CHANGING YOUR OIL IS MORE DIFFICULT THAN YOU THOUGHT

	% Linoleic Acid	% Linolenic Acid	% Oleic Acid	% Saturated Fats
Flaxseed (linseed)	15	54	20	9
Pumpkin seed	45	15	29	8
Soybean	42	11	31	15
Walnut	50	5	28	16
Canola	26	8	54	9
Almond	17		67	15
Virgin Olive	12		68	16
Safflower	70		15	12
Sunflower	66		22	12
Corn	59		25	13
Sesame	45		41	17
Rice bran	35		48	17

The Oleic Acid Story

Why has there been so much mention of olive oil as the oil of choice for longevity? It contains only one of the essential oils (linoleic acid) and not linolenic acid.

In 1987, experiments showed that diets rich in olive oil lower total cholesterol but do not lower the "good" cholesterol. In 1988, another study showed that diets rich in olive oil also lowered the "bad" cholesterol.

Then in 1990, Dr. David Steenblock and his crew at the University of California, San Diego, showed that oleic acid was able to block the oxidation of "bad" cholesterol before it could damage arteries. (More about antioxidants later on.)

So, olive oil (virgin olive oil) gives your body a healthful combination of linoleic and oleic acids. While some of the other oils also provide healthful combinations, not all of them lend themselves to the variety of cooking and salad techniques that olive oil does.

In one respect, olive oil is no different from other culinary oils. There's 120 calories per tablespoon, but it can help lower bad cholesterol and maintain good cholesterol.

Olives are pressed once and the oil is then tested for flavor and acidity. The highest quality, extra virgin, is a dark yellow to green oil with a fragrant, full-bodied taste and a hefty price tag. It can run from $8 to $30 a liter (1 qt., 2 fl. oz.).

Since it loses its flavor if heated, such as in sautéing, the extra virgin oil is best when used straight out of the bottle. Drizzle it over fresh vegetables, cooked vegetables or salads.

Oil that doesn't qualify as extra virgin is processed to lower acidity and reduce bitterness. The processing removes color and flavor so the producers spike it by adding up to 30 percent extra virgin oil. The result is labeled "pure olive oil" or "olive oil" and at $5 to $8 a liter, makes a good all-purpose oil, well suited for sautéing.

"Light" olive oil is made for the U.S. market. It's pure olive oil but with less than 5 percent extra virgin. It's called light only because of its milder taste, but the calories and health benefits are the same. The light olive oil is recommended for baking since it does not add any taste to your recipe.

Many stores have a wide variety of oils and brands. If you can find a good Italian grocery you can ask for advice about the best oil for your eating purposes.

In addition to olive (or similar) oil, eat fatty fish three times a week, use fish oil supplements and a capsule of gamma-linolenic acid twice a day, and you've begun your "live to be 100" campaign.

However, there are still other things you have to do. Read on.

Anti-aging Antioxidants

It is really important to understand that aging and disease are two different things.

Aging is that mysterious process that leads to death.

Disease is usually the result of individual lifestyle.

It is logical that we can slow the aging process by staying healthy and preventing disease.

Despite the hundreds of different medical terms that are used to describe them, many aging processes, and most diseased conditions, are nothing more than an accumulation of cellular damage. *In these situations, more cells are being damaged than the body is able to repair or replace.*

The understanding of this concept and its implications is overwhelming when we realize that much of this cellular damage has its beginning or ending in a free-radical-induced chemical reaction.

When the levels of free radicals are greater than the supply of antioxidant enzymes, we speak of free radical pathology which represents a more accurate definition of the cause of most conditions than the current terms being used, which tend to denote the result (i.e. cancer, heart disease, etc.). (Figure 1)

Additionally, free radical damage to certain types of cells is irreversible. Three types of cells: heart muscle cells, nerve cells (which include brain cells), and certain sensor cells of the immune system cannot be replaced in the adult human. Damage to these types of cells must be prevented to ensure a long and healthy life.

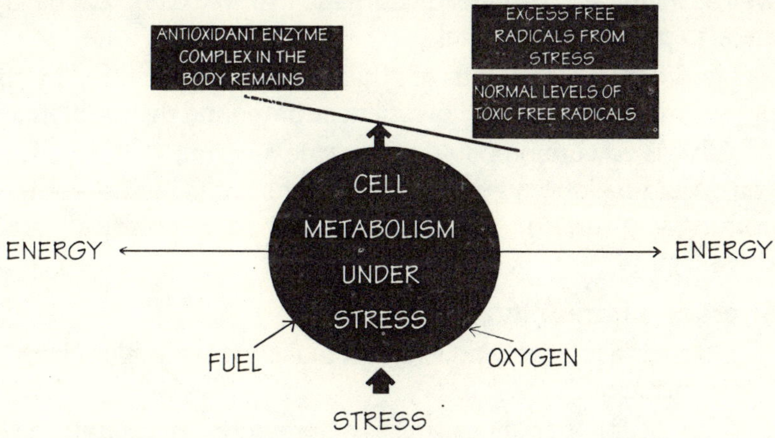

FIGURE 1
Excess free radicals from stress create imbalance and free radical pathology.

Once again, this is not to imply that excess free radical activity is the sole cause of aging or disease. Yet, it is true that a large majority of unnecessary cellular damage which leads to aging and disease can be avoided by following two simple guidelines.

First, the free radical causing stress in our lives must be reduced or removed.

Second, the antioxidant enzyme, or anti-free radical defense system of the body must be properly supported. *If even one of these premises can be implemented effectively, the process of our own individual aging or disease potential will be altered significantly.*

The unfortunate truth is that many forms of free-radical-causing stress that originate in our so-called civilized environment and society are completely unavoidable.

For example, while it is true that it is entirely up to you to give up smoking, drinking and eating junk food, you'll find it very difficult to avoid inhaling polluted air — especially if you live in the city.

Pesticide residues on food and in water are also difficult to avoid completely. Radioactive wastes and nuclear experiments, as well as increased cosmic radiation due to a weakened ozone layer, are also potentially harmful.

Additionally, hundreds of other force fields generated by computers, microwaves, and power lines compound the problem.

Unless you are prepared to become a hermit — in which case you would have to adjust to a different set of stresses — there is nothing you can do to eliminate all of these free-radical-causing stress factors.

Stress and Immunity

Stress is a relatively new notion that everybody talks about, yet few understand.

The dictionary defines stress as "pressure, force, strain: a state of physical or mental tension inducing it, or affecting something." This definition, while obviously correct, is not very helpful in understanding the concept of stress.

On the other hand, it is important to comprehend the notion, because all of us are continuously exposed to stress.

Stress occurs in many forms. The four major categories which concern us are:

1. Chemical stress
2. Emotional stress
3. Physical trauma
4. Infections

Each of these stress forms can originate from multiple sources. Most of these have appeared as primary threats in our environment as recently as this century.

For example, chemical stress can come from pesticides, insecticides, polluted air and water, heavy metals such as mercury or lead, asbestos and, worst of all, radioactive waste.

Even jet travel, a welcome commonplace today but unheard of a mere half a century ago, exposes passengers to unhealthy high levels of ozone and random cosmic radiations.

In the light of such widespread physiological insult, it is a true miracle that any of us manage to stay healthy at all.

One of the primary reasons why stress is so important to understand is because it is intricately linked to the functioning of our immune systems.

How have many of us have gotten a cold when our defenses were impaired by excessive stress? This is another angle from which to view the recent rash of immune disorders unleashed in our culture. Could these problems be partly caused by an overwhelmed immune system? It should be obvious that this is quite possible, and the more we consider the high levels of stress that most of us are exposed to daily, the more relevant the idea becomes.

In other words, understanding and compensating for the stress in our lives will help our immune systems and enhance our ability to stay well.

This is not to imply that all stress is harmful. Exercise, for example, is a form of stress on the body which is quite healthy. Yet, if we over-exert ourselves during exercise, we can damage the body and create problems.

As we have already mentioned, many unavoidable stress factors, such as pollution, and others that cause damage to the body, stem from today's world of technological progress. In many cases the physical result brought on by several different forms of stress is the same. *These unnecessary, but avoidable, results are cellular damage caused by overactive molecules called free radicals.*

Target Nutrients for Pollution Defense—Antioxidants

A perfect diet is not enough. Certain vitamins, minerals, and herbs not only replace nutrients robbed by pollutants, they can also reinforce our immune system, defending us against harmful chemicals.

The *antioxidant* vitamins and minerals and specific detoxifying herbs are the target nutrients for pollution defense. What has been called controlled oxidation is a natural part of metabolism. The burning of the body's fuel is oxidation at work. However, the pollutants we breathe, eat and absorb (including environmental pollutants like pollen, dust, and mold) are converted by enzymes into a new molecular form called free radicals. These cause uncontrolled oxidation, and have been implicated in cancer, heart diseases and serious infectious diseases as well as hypersensitivities or environmental illnesses. Internal pollution, including smoking, consumption of caffeine, alcohol and drugs, plus stress, all increase free radical activity in the body.

Vitamins — C, E, A, beta-carotene and the minerals selenium and zinc are the most important antioxidants. They protect the cell from damage by preventing the combining of free radicals with cell components. Greater intake of vitamins C and E along with iron and calcium will reduce the risk of lead absorption and accumulation.

Vitamin C — Shown to interact with over 50 pollutants, including those categorized as pesticides, heavy metals, selected hydrocarbons and gaseous pollutants. It is the most effective defense against the cancer-causing compounds formed from the nitrites and nitrates used to color and preserve cured meats and other processed foods. One study at MIT showed that a total of 2,000 mg of C successfully blocked nitrosamine formation. Vitamin C is far stronger than any medicine and far faster, with no side effects at all. Take vitamin C supplements (about 1-3 grams per day).

Vitamin E — Best known for its ability to protect against cigarette smoke inhalation, it can also prevent the formation of free radicals by oxygen, ozone, nitrogen dioxide and the sun's rays. Researchers from the University of Kentucky and California exposed rats to the deadly air pollutant ozone (not the same as the protective ozone of the earth's atmosphere). The groups which had been fed a diet rich in vitamin E "emerged unscathed." Supplement recommendations range from 90-800 IU/day.

Vitamin A — Counters pollutants that stress our lungs. Bacteria, poisonous gases, and other airborne pollutants kill epithelial cells that line the respiratory tract. With sufficient vitamin A these cells have the power to regenerate themselves, protecting the body from upper respiratory infection and lung disease (5000 IU/d).

Beta-Carotene — The substance that gives yellow color to fruits and vegetables, it works as a precursor to vitamin A. However, it functions in the body like vitamin E, working in the cell membrane. Beta-carotene is associated with lowered cancer risk, and unlike vitamin A, large amounts have negligible toxicity.

Minerals — Zinc, copper, manganese, selenium, and iron. These are the crucial components of the antioxidant enzymes. Because of their effectiveness, these enzymes are considered the first line of defense against free radicals. The antioxidant enzymes, such as superoxide dismutase (SOD), glutathione peroxidase, and catalase, each need a particular mineral to do their job. Zinc is especially important and has been linked to human immune deficiency.

Amino Acids — Methionine, cysteine, taurine: These sulfur-bearing aminos are essential to the formation of glutathione, an important water-bearing antioxidant. Methionine is an essential amino acid which means we must eat foods that contain it because it cannot be synthesized by our bodies. However, both cysteine and taurine can be synthesized if methionine is present.

Coenzyme Q-10 — CoQ is needed by the body for the production of energy. In its capacity as an antioxidant, it is found in the lipid membranes like vitamin E and beta-carotene.

Gamma-linolenic acid (GLA) — GLA is a key regulator of T-lymphocyte function in the body. GLA can be made from linoleic acid, which is found in vegetable oils, but if magnesium, zinc, vitamin C, B^6, B^3, and A are not present in sufficient amounts, the conversion may be blocked.

Pycnogenol — This remarkable plant-derived substance is a blend of special bioflavonoids with potent antioxidant activity. It is said to reduce free radical damage even more effectively than vitamin E, to potentiate the health-giving effects of vitamin C, and protect brain and nerve tissue because it easily passes through the blood-brain barrier. More about this powerful antioxidant further on.

You've Read About Beta-carotene, But Have You Heard About Its Cousin Alpha-carotene?

Where does the color of your foods come from?

The color and the health benefits come from about 500 phytochemicals called carotenoids. The most publicized of them has been beta-carotene with its wonderful health-protecting power of preventing and, in some cases, reversing cancer!

Can we do even better?

How about another carotenoid, perhaps ten times as protective of your body. It's called alpha-carotene. The discovery of this phytochemical was done by Michiaki Murakoshi et al., at the Kyoto Prefectual University, Japan. He reported that alpha-carotene suppressed the growth of several types of malignant tumors, including pancreatic cancer and gastric cancer. This was reported in the *Journal of the National Cancer Institute* (Nov. 1, 1989; 81: 1649-52). Alpha-carotene began working against cancer cells after just 8 hours and many of those cells reversed and began normal activity. The higher the dose, the greater the benefits.

In follow-up studies it was also found that it was more effective than beta-carotene against liver, lung, and skin cancers. Alpha-carotene, when not immediately needed, is stored in your liver. Perhaps it is also protective of that very important organ while it sits and waits for something nasty to show up.

And still more about phytochemicals like carotenoids. Although we've discovered beta-carotene and alpha-carotene, and have began to understand their power, there's gamma-carotene on the horizon.

Wouldn't it be wonderful if antibiotics were no longer needed?

Alpha-carotene is now available at health food stores. Follow label directions.

While you're in the store, look for a new rival to vitamin E. Vitamin E is a wonderful antioxidant and should be a part of every supplement program, up to 800 I.U. daily; but a new phytochemical derived from — of all things — palm oil, has 100 times the biological power of vitamin E. In *Archives of Biochemistry and Biophysics* (Nov. 1, 1989; 532-8), it was first reported that a substance called Lycopene was one of the best dietary antioxidants. However, the research wasn't followed up at that time.

When your mother said to eat a lot of color foods, she really knew what she was talking about.

Future Roles for Vitamins in Disease Prevention

Presented at the Antioxidant Vitamin and Beta-Carotene in Disease Prevention Conference:

Eating foods rich in vitamins could offset the diseases of old age and protect the lungs against damaging effects of smog and cigarette smoke, scientists announced at this conference. *But nutritional analyses suggest the average diet of people in many countries is likely to be seriously short of the necessary vitamins.*

Research findings backing claims for health benefits attributed to diets rich in vitamins C and E and beta-carotene were presented at the conference held in London.

U.S. expert Dr. Richard Cutler of the Gerontology Research Center, Baltimore, said there is now a great deal of experimental evidence showing that oxygen free radicals are an important part of the aging process. The implications of this research suggest that people who increase the concentration of antioxidant substances in their body tissues will age more slowly and delay the onset of diseases associated with old age. These substances are the vitamins C and E as well as beta-carotene.

Professor William Pryor of Louisiana State University said *supplementing the diet with vitamin E over* the long term could protect against damage from ozone present in smog.

Oxidation caused by ozone in smog can damage the immune system. People breathing ozone-contaminated air can therefore be expected to be more susceptible to infectious diseases.

As Professor Pryor pointed out, vitamin E appears to enhance the immune system, particularly after long term therapy. It is quite likely, therefore, that *supplementing the diet with vitamin E* on a long term basis would protect against ozone-induced weakening of the immune system. The anti-cancer properties of vitamin E might similarly protect against smog-induced tumors.

Research presented by Professor Ronald Anderson of Pretoria University, South Africa, showed that administering high levels of vitamin E and beta-carotene to smokers could reduce the amount of smoke-induced toxic free radicals which impair respiratory function.

A major effort is needed to stress to the public the importance of increasing the amount of fruit and vegetables (sources of antioxidant vitamins C and A) in the diet, U.S. cancer epidemiologist Dr. Gladys Block told the conference.

Despite the recommendations of the U.S. National Academy of Sciences that people should consume five or more servings of fruit and vegetables daily, Dr. Block said there was evidence that few Americans ate anything like this quantity. Almost half of those surveyed in a 24-hour dietary recall study ate no fruit at all and less than a third had eaten a fruit rich in vitamin C. Other countries are likely to find a similar situation, said Dr. Block.

Note: The servings of fruits and vegetables recommended here would provide significant amounts of vitamins A and C — but not vitamin E. Vitamin E is present in nuts, whole grains, and oils. The average American diet is estimated to provide only 10.4-13.4 IU — largely because vitamin E is destroyed in food processing and because weight-conscious individuals cut down on the calorie-rich foods that contain vitamin E.

To get as much vitamin E as is contained in a 400 IU supplement capsule, you would have to eat 1 pound of sunflower seeds, more than 5 pounds of wheat germ, or 2 quarts of corn oil a day. This is equivalent to as much as 8000 calories. For this reason, those who wish to ensure that they are getting enough vitamin E to provide antioxidant protection should use a supplement.

It's Not What Cholesterol Does to You But What You Do to Cholesterol

Of course, you should control your fat and cholesterol intake, for all the multitude of reasons science has laid out in the medical journals, the popular press, radio and T.V.

But, a radical, new concept is changing our perception of what happens to the cholesterol once it's in our body.

After all, our liver manufactures cholesterol.

Is it good or bad cholesterol we manufacture?

If we don't get enough cholesterol from the food we eat, the liver makes enough to make up the difference!

If we ate a completely fat-free, cholesterol free diet, we'd die.

Welcome to the new world of cholesterol and life extension, and what happens to cholesterol when it's attacked by those dangerous free radicals.

"Free radicals are great white sharks in the biochemical sea."

Roy Walford, M.D.
Maximum Life Span (Avon, 1983)

"When there is excessive oxidation and a deficiency of antioxidants, the excess free radicals are free to create havoc in the body. They are involved in aging, immune disease, cancer, and, of course, in chemical sensitivities and allergies."

Abram Hoffer, M.D., Ph.D.

". . . a provocative theory linking vitamin consumption to protection from heart disease is holding up and gathering strength."

". . . how can cholesterol, a substance that is a constituent of every cell's membrane and that is completely inert when mixed with cells in the laboratory, elicit bumps and lesions on the slick linings of artery walls?"

". . . basic research said that the answer lay in oxidation: cholesterol must be oxidized, made rancid, before it does damage."

The New York Times
September 22, 1992

The relationship among free radicals, antioxidants, tumors, cancers, radiation, chemical pollutants, and aging is still a new and provocative subject area. "Free radical pathology is as great a breakthrough in medicine as Pasteur's germ theory of disease."

Harry Demopoulos, M.D.
New York University School of Medicine
Department of Pathology

Reduced severity of atherosclerosis (and in some cases, even regression of arterial blockage) in primates after supplementation with natural vitamin E was reported this week by A.J. Verlangieri, Ph.D., and M.J. Bush of the Atherosclerosis Research Laboratory at the University of Mississippi. In the April issue of the *Journal of the American College of Nutrition,* the researchers concluded that natural vitamin E may be effective in lessening the severity and reducing the rate of incidence of atherosclerosis. The animals were supplemented at eight times the daily requirement for the species.

The American Cancer Society announced a policy shift and will focus major resources on preventing cancer through dietary modification because of new nutrition research findings.

At the recent meeting of the New York Academy of Sciences, Ishwarial Jialal, M.D., of the University of Texas, Southwestern Medical Center in Dallas, reported that antioxidant nutrients may be instrumental in preventing heart disease by suppressing the oxidation of certain fat particles (low density lipoproteins — LDL's) in the bloodstream.

Dr. Jialal stated that in his studies "vitamin C, vitamin E and beta-carotene all inhibited LDL oxidation and the early stages of plaque formation."

According to several studies by Charles H. Hennekens, M.D., of the Harvard Medical School in Boston, the antioxidant nutrients also appear to reduce heart disease risk. Dr. Hennekens found that men and women who consume high levels of beta-carotene and vitamin E from foods had fewer heart attacks, strokes and deaths related to heart disease than those who consume less of these two antioxidants.

Simin N. Meydani, D.V.M., Ph.D., of the USDA Human Nutrition Research Center on Aging, reported that vitamins E and B^6 play an important role in maintenance of the body's immune response, its system for fighting infection and disease. "The elderly may need supplementation of vitamins E and B^6 at levels higher than the RDA to maintain optimal immunity," said Dr. Meydani.

The Times
Thursday, October 5, 1989
International Health Conference, Westminster, England.

Speakers from research centers around the world claimed that foods containing antioxidant vitamins could protect the public from developing cancer and might also slow down the growth of early tumors. The long list of other beneficial effects included protection against heart disease, cataracts and the effects of smoking, the delaying of aging and slowing the progress of Parkinson's disease.

The vitamins for which the greatest claims are being made are the antioxidants vitamin C, E, and beta-carotene.

The Times
October 3, 1989

Professor Anthony Diplock, head of biochemistry at Guy's and St. Thomas's Hospitals, Central London, said there was growing evidence to support the free radical theory of disease and the protective role of vitamins and carotenoids as antioxidants. If the body's level of antioxidants is low, free radicals proliferate and cause damage.

Convincing evidence has emerged for the protective role of vitamin E in cancer and heart disease.

The Daily Telegraph
Tuesday, October 3, 1989

Dr. William Pryor, Professor of Chemistry and Biochemistry at Louisiana State University said there was increasing evidence of the role of vitamins C and E and beta-carotene, a nutrient found mainly in yellow and orange fruits and vegetables, in protecting against disease.

Asked whether increased consumption of vegetables supplemented with vitamins would prolong life, Prof. Pryor said: "You don't retard aging by taking vitamins but you do retard the onset of the chronic killer diseases which has the effect of lengthening the lifespan of the population."

Today
October 3, 1989

Professor William Pryor, Head of Biochemistry at Louisiana University, suggested that people eat a balanced diet and take supplemental vitamins. "The evidence is that vitamins are beneficial. Their toxicity is virtually zero. They are known to be safe."

The New York Times
Tuesday, March 10, 1992

Researchers are gathering provocative evidence that vitamins influence the health and vibrancy of nearly every organ, and that these enigmatic chemicals may help forestall or even reverse many diseases of aging, including cancer, heart disease, osteoporosis, a flagging immune system, neurodegeneration and other chronic diseases.

FIRST BIG STUDY FINDS THAT VITAMIN SUPPLEMENTS CUT CANCER DEATHS

(*The New York Times,* Wednesday, September 15, 1993)

While the FDA and the AMA follow a pattern of avoidance and denial as they campaign against a free flow of supplements, a report published in the *Journal of the National Cancer Institute,* Wednesday, September 15, 1993, states that they have evidence from a large human study that vitamin supplementation could reduce the risk of cancer.

The study of nearly 30,000 residents of an area of north-central China where cancer death rates are among the highest in the world showed that nutritional supplements could reduce the risk of dying from cancer and other diseases.

The research team was made up of both Chinese and American scientists who conducted the study over a five year period. Residents of Linxian County in the Henan Province were given either a dummy pill or a combination of supplements including vitamin E, selenium and beta-carotene.

The results, among those fortunate enough to have received the vitamins, showed an overall drop in cancer deaths by 13% and a drop in the risk of death from other causes by almost 10%.

Dr. Peter Greenwald, director of the cancer institute's division of cancer prevention and control, said that several major studies were under way in the U.S. to see if vitamin-mineral supplements could prevent cancer, but that conclusive results were years away. Do you want to wait for the results?

Antioxidants Are News

Not a magic elixir. . . not a secret formula handed down through the ages, but enzymes, vitamins, minerals, and accessory nutrients found in foods and used as supplements.

Why?

Because recent research into free radicals — tiny, reactive molecules made during normal metabolism and found in increasingly larger amounts in our polluted world — suggests they can do the kinds of damage that leads to heart disease, cancer, brain disorders, and a host of degenerative diseases including aging.

How Can Those Tiny, Free Radical Molecules Hurt Us?

Free radicals are unbalanced. Not unbalanced crazy, but unbalanced because they have an odd number of electrons in their outermost orbit and either have to rape a neighboring molecule and steal an electron for balancing, or shoot off one electron like a bullet into another molecule which satisfies the original free radical but plunges that other molecule into the unstable, unbalanced situation.

What Does That Do?

It sets off a chain reaction involving thousands of molecules. It's the kind of damage that occurs when butter turns rancid. Can you image what could happen to you if the fat in your body began to turn rancid? Chemical changes inside living cells can cause genetic mutations, alter the structure of important proteins, disable fatty molecules, and more.

In the Beginning

The earliest life on earth was anaerobic. It had to be so because there was no oxygen present in the atmosphere. Energy production in the early forms of life was through a fermentation process. After the passage of time, more advanced organisms utilized solar energy in photosynthesis and released oxygen as a by-product. Over eons, this release of oxygen gradually transformed the atmosphere from anaerobic to aerobic (oxygen containing). With this transformation, organisms evolved that were adapted to the oxygen environment, eventually utilizing oxygen in respiration to generate great amounts of energy.

Those organisms eventually became you and I, and the process of utilizing oxygen is called oxidation.

This controlled oxidation that occurs in respiration is an efficient energy-producing system. However, it is not a fail-proof system since, along with energy, the respiratory-metabolic activity also produces unstable oxygen by-products called free radicals.

Free radicals are capable of damaging DNA, proteins, carbohydrates, and lipids. The process of free radical oxidation is familiar to all of us since we see it in the rusting of metal, the browning of fruit and the rancidity of oils.

In addition to the generation of free radicals internally, they are also generated in the atmosphere as by-products of radiation, pollution, cigarette smoke, sunlight, and herbicides.

There are five basic types of damage caused by free radicals:

1. Lipid peroxidation, in which free radicals initiate damage to fat compounds in the body, causing them to turn rancid and release more free radicals. It is their action upon cholesterol that makes that substance dangerous to health.
2. Cross-linking, in which free-radical reactions cause proteins and/or DNA molecules to fuse together.
3. Membrane damage, in which free-radical reactions destroy the integrity of the cell membranes, which in turn interfere with the cell's ability to take in nutrients and expel waste material.
4. Lysosome damage, in which free-radical reactions rupture the cell's digestive particle membrane inside the cell, which then spills the contents into the cell and digests critical cell components. The cell literally "eats" itself alive.
5. Accumulation of lipofuscin (age pigment) which can interfere with cell chemistry. It is lipofuscin which causes those ugly brown spots on your hands. Those same accumulations occur in other, internal areas as a result of free-radical intrusion.

The most damaging agents of free-radical reactions include the superoxide, hydroxyl, and lipid peroxide radicals and hydrogen peroxide.

The Antioxidant Defense System

Nature is no fool!

We weren't put on this earth to be wiped out by free radicals without a fight. To control the free radicals, an elaborate system of antioxidants has evolved that can protect our cells' organs and tissues against the oxidative threats. All aerobic organisms, animal and human, share this "pollution control" system. The health or disease of each cell and each tissue depends on the balance between its antioxidant protection and its proxidant components.

Our armament includes these "heavy hitters" among our major biological antioxidants:

ANTIOXIDANT ENZYMES
Superoxide dismutase (SOD)
Catalase
Glutathione peroxidase

ANTIOXIDANT NUTRIENTS
Vitamin C
Vitamin E
Vitamin A
Alpha-carotene
Beta-carotene
Selenium
Zinc
L-cysteine
L-methionine
Pycnogenol
Polyphenols
Bioflavonoids
Coenzyme Q-10
Ginkgo biloba
Gamma-linolenic acid (GLA)

The antioxidants often work synergistically. The body army sends different antioxidant "patrols" out into various biological territories. The antioxidant enzymes and vitamins are strategically placed within the cell to guard the cell's internal structure. Antioxidant vitamins can also circulate freely in the blood and neutralize free radicals outside the cell.

Vitamin E, the powerful fat-soluble antioxidant guardian lodges both within the membranes inside and the membranes surrounding the cell, strengthening the cell against a free radical attack. It also protects one of its partners, beta-carotene, from being attacked.

Vitamin C, a water-soluble soldier, interacts with free radicals in the water, in cells and in intercellular fluids. In addition, vitamin C can "recycle" vitamin E by regenerating it chemically after it has been spent in terminating a free radical reaction.

Beta-carotene inactivates singlet oxygen, a fiercely active form of oxygen often generated by exposure to sunlight. Because of this ability, it has a photo-protective effect in the skin against ultraviolet light.

ANTIOXIDANT ACTIVITY OF BETA-CAROTENE

$$O_2 + (e-) \rightarrow \bullet O_2$$

(superoxide amion radical)

$$\bullet O_2- + (e-) + 2H+ \rightarrow H_2O_2$$

(hydrogen peroxide)

$$H_2O_2 + (e-) + H+ \rightarrow H_2O + HO\bullet$$

(hydroxyl radical)

$$HO\bullet + (e-) + H+ \rightarrow H_2O$$

Source: Levine (with Kidd), The Biochemistry of Free Radicals. In: *Antioxidant Adaptation: Its Role in Free Radical Pathology,* Biocurrents Division, Allergy Research Group: San Leandro CA. p10 (1985)

The body can split a molecule of beta-carotene in half to form two molecules of vitamin A. But beta-carotene is more than just a precursor of vitamin A, it has its own chemistry independent of vitamin A chemistry. Thus, beta-carotene can offer the protection of vitamin A plus all of its activity as a whole molecule. Therefore, the inclusion of beta-carotene-containing foods or beta-carotene supplements into your daily regimen serves a double purpose.

A Perfect Diet May Not Be Enough, But it Helps!

Food choices play a key role in increasing our chances of avoiding certain physical and mental disasters. However, can we get enough of the antioxidants we need from food alone? Most nutritional scientists are in agreement that diet alone cannot supply all the protection we need in this highly polluted environment we call our neighborhood, but eating foods high in protective nutrients will give our bodies a head start.

The Protectors

These are the foods highest in vitamins A and C and the mineral selenium.

FOOD	PORTION	VITAMIN A (I.U.)	VITAMIN C (MGS.)	SELENIUM (MCGS.)
Beef kidneys	3 oz.	846	0	132
Beef liver	3 oz.	45,390	23	37
Beet greens	1 cup	7,400	22	
Bran flakes	1 cup	1,540	0	*
Broccoli	1 stalk	4,500	162	*
Cantaloupe	1/2 melon	9,240	90	
Carrots, raw	1 medium	7,930	6	
Chinese cabbage	1 cup	5,270	26	
Cod	3 oz.	150	0	27
Collard greens	1 cup	14,820	144	
Corn flakes	1 cup	1,760	21	
Oranges	1 medium	260	66	
Orange juice	1 cup	540	120	
Oysters	13 to 19	740	0	157
Pumpkin, canned	1 cup	15,680	12	
Soup, vegetarian	1 cup	2,940	0	
Spinach	1 cup	14,580	50	
Squash, winter	1 cup	8,610	27	
Sweet potatoes	1 medium	9,230	25	
Tomatoes	1 medium	1,110	28	*
Tomatoes, canned	1 cup	2,170	41	*
Watermelon	1 wedge	2,510	30	

NOTE: An asterisk (*) indicates that the food contains selenium, but the amount is not yet known. Assume all fruits are raw and other foods cooked unless otherwise noted. Chart compiled with the help of the USDA.

Here's How To Get the Beta-carotene You Need:

The Winners (more than 1,000 IUs per serving):

Apricots, broccoli, cantaloupe, carrots, dark-green leafy vegetables; spinach, turnip greens, kale, etc. (romaine lettuce, but not iceberg lettuce), mangoes, peaches, pumpkins, squash (winter), sweet potatoes.

Honorable Mention (500-1,000 IUs per serving):

Asparagus, brussels sprouts, green beans, peas, squash (summer), tomatoes, watermelon.

The Recommendation: At least two servings of foods high in beta carotene every day.

Here's How To Get the Other Nutrients You Need:

Vitamin E: Vegetable oils, margarine, wheat germ, whole-grain cereal and bread, dried beans, green leafy vegetables.

Zinc: Poultry, seafood, milk, liver, red meat, whole grains.

Selenium: Seafood, whole-grain cereals, red meat, egg yolk, chicken, milk, garlic.

The Recommendation: Include the above foods in a balanced diet low in fats, high in complex carbohydrates.

Getting Older Without Aging

Chromium is a trace mineral required by our bodies in minute amounts. You need about 200 micrograms daily of this essential mineral.

What's a microgram?

One-millionth of a gram. Obviously, a very tiny amount but if we didn't supply it to our body we couldn't live.

Chromium levels are highest in young people in their teens and twenties and decline progressively with each succeeding decade. It is the only mineral to show a continuing decrease with age.

Any form of stress can deplete already small chromium stores. Exercise (good stress), emotional trauma, pollution, cold weather, modern living (bad stress) acts to use up chromium.

So, take a chromium picolinate supplement, 200 mcg daily. Ignore the nay-sayers who tell you that chromium is a poison. Yes, the chromium used on your car's bumper is poisonous but it is hexavalent chromium. The chromium in your supplement is trivalent, and about as poisonous as a glass of water.

Suggestions to Reduce Calorie and Fat Intake and Help You to Live a Longer Life

Suggestion #1

Control your calorie and fat intake.

There are many ways to cut down on calories, carbohydrates and fats without ever feeling deprived. Try some of the following exchanges.

Instead of:	*Try this:*
Cookies	Rice cakes
Nuts	Popcorn
Deviled eggs	Stuff the whites with tuna or shrimp salad
Steak tidbits	Chicken tidbits
Salad dressing	Lemon juice or vinegar with a touch of cooking oil
Cream sauce for vegetables	Low-cal dressings or bouillon
Ground beef for meat loaf	Fresh ground turkey
Beef or pork hot dogs	Hot dogs from chicken or turkey
Mayonnaise	Low-cal mayonnaise
Pasta meat sauce	Instant soup mixes to flavor
Gin and tonic	Club soda or seltzer with twist of lemon or lime
Sour cream	Plain unflavored yogurt
Cream of chicken soup	Chicken broth
Orange juice punch	Tomato juice punch
Sugary sauces or catsup	Herbs such as onion, garlic for flavoring peppers, horseradish, soy sauce, ginger, basil

Instead of:	*Try this:*
Fruit-flavored liqueurs	Fruit juices and dash of brandy extract
Chocolate	Carob powder (less bitter, so needs less sweetener); for stronger chocolate taste, add instant coffee and dash of vanilla.
Catsup	Tomato puree or tomato juice
Tartar sauce	Mix low-cal mayonnaise with dill pickle relish or lemon juice
Sugar in pie recipes	Increase fruit or raisins
Fruit packed in syrup	Packed in water or natural juice
Hollandaise sauce	Low-fat mayonnaise thinned with boiling water, dash of lemon, cayenne
Thickening with flour	Cornstarch or arrowroot
Coconut milk for flavor	Coconut extract or grated coconut
Coconut or palm cooking oil	Corn, olive or soybean oil
Processed cheese dip	Low-cal cottage cheese plus herbs
Sardines	Shrimp, boiled
Pecans	Black or English walnuts
Cashew nuts	Sunflower seeds
Mayonnaise in tuna salad	Unsweetened low-fat yogurt and seasoning
Cracker crumbs in meatballs	Wheat bran
Sweet barbecue sauce	Tomato paste and herbs
Sugar and flour cake	Thick watermelon covered with grapes, strawberries, raspberries

Instead of:	*Try this:*
Avocado in salad	Mung, alfalfa or bean sprouts
Coffee creamer of coconut oil	Creamer made from soybean oil or evaporated skimmed milk
Prime cut of beef with marbling	Choice or ungraded, less marbling
Gourmet ice cream	Non-gourmet (half as much fat)
Ice cream	Ice milk, frozen low-fat yogurt
Fried chicken	Lemon baked chicken
Scalloped potatoes with cheese	Baked potato with chives
Fried zucchini	Steamed zucchini
Apple pie	Baked apple with cinnamon
Strawberry shortcake	Fresh strawberries
Ricotta cheese topping	Tofu (bean curd)
Fish, breaded and fried	Fish, broiled
Fried egg	Poached or boiled egg
Peanuts	Raw carrots, celery sticks, pickles
Cocktail	Cranberry or orange juice and ice
Sugar-coated cereal	No-sugar shredded wheat, oats
Chocolate chip cookies	No-sugar fruit and oats cookie

You can reduce fat in your diet rather simply. Eat more salads, vegetables and grains, avoid gravies and rich sauces, drink less whole milk, eat less meat and more fish and poultry, avoid fried foods.

Also watch for hidden fats. It isn't just sugar that is bad in cakes, cookies, doughnuts, ice cream and candy.

You don't have to give up eggs. If your cholesterol level is too high, you can limit your intake to two or three a week. If your level is normal, then eat lots of eggs — they are very nutritious.

Drink lots of water.

Use non-fattening methods of cooking.

Limit alcohol consumption. Beer contains chromium but no more than one glass of beer a day.

Limit your intake of sodium and sugar.

Limit highly refined or highly processed foods.

Eat fresh foods whenever possible.

Follow the nutritional supplement program suggested in this section of the book.

Suggestion #2

Use lipotropics in your supplement program.

Lipotropics play important roles in a protective fat metabolism program. They are nutrients which enable the body to handle fats efficiently. They stimulate the production of special types of fats called phospholipids found in the membranes of all body tissues. Phospholipids have an emulsifying action on triglycerides (the storage form of fat stored in adipose tissue and the blood) and cholesterol. They act like nature's soap: they break up insoluble deposits of fats and cholesterol, converting them to small suspended globules which can be washed away in the bloodstream. High-density lipoprotein (HDL), the good cholesterol, is composed mostly of these phospholipid "soups".

The two most commonly used lipotropes are choline and inositol (known as phosphatidyl choline and phosphatidyl inositol). They are frequently found in lipotropic formulas found in health food stores along with methionine (an amino acid).

Take a lipotropic formula daily according to label directions. Or — take a supplement of phosphatidyl choline daily, according to label instructions.

Or — take two capsules of lecithin with each meal.

Suggestion #3

Supplementary intake of L-carnitine will provide important health benefits on the road to 100.

The biochemical role of L-carnitine is to enable fats to be transported into the cells so they can be burned as a source of energy.

Stands to reason that if there's not enough L-carnitine floating around to yank the fats from the bloodstream and feed them into the cell's furnace, the fats can build up in the blood.

Studies indicate that using supplements of L-carnitine can lower blood fat levels and stimulate fat-burning. So, not only do you get lower fat levels in your blood, but you may lose some stored fat besides.

Also, L-carnitine can offer cardiovascular protection by minimizing the toxic effect of fat on oxygen-deprived heart tissue.

Take L-carnitine 100 to 300 mg daily. Available from your health food store.

Suggestion #4

The Nutritional Antioxidants

We've discussed in detail the effect of oxidation on cholesterol. Antioxidants can mean the difference in the race to achieve 100 years. Most vitamin/mineral formulas will supply an adequate amount of the B-complex vitamins, most of the essential minerals, and enough vitamins A and D. However, you will have to take additional supplements to round out your antioxidant levels, as well as minerals needed in larger than trace amounts such as calcium, magnesium combinations.

How much should you take?

We'll have to turn to the animals to try to get an idea of what would be ideal for a human. Most creatures in the world make their own vitamin C. Humans can't manufacture this important vitamin because we lost the ability some 65,000 years ago. But if we take animals and compare the weight (which approximates the number of cells in the body), we should arrive at a correct amount. Using an average human weight of 132 pounds, an animal of the same weight would make this much vitamin C for itself every day:

- one 132 pound toad would make 11 grams of vitamin C
- one 132 pound frog would make 9 grams of vitamin C
- one 132 pound goat would make 5 grams of vitamin C
- one 132 pound cow would make 4 grams of vitamin C
- one 132 pound rabbit would make 2 grams of vitamin C

If we place humans somewhere between a rabbit and a frog, we'd probably arrive at the same daily amounts figured out by Dr. M. Colgan of the Colgan Institute, one of the foremost institutions devoted to nutritional research. Based on his research and animal studies, these are the daily amounts of antioxidants that may maintain a protective shield.

Vitamin C*	2000 – 12,000 mg
Vitamin E	400 – 800 I.U.
Selenium	200 – 400 mcg
L-glutathione	50 – 250 mg
Zinc	20 – 70 mg
Coenzyme Q-10	30 – 60 mg
Beta carotene	5000 – 25,000 I.U.

You will also have to get separate supplements of ginkgo biloba and pycnogenol from your health food store (follow label directions). The same with calcium (1000 to 1500 mg) and magnesium (500 to 750 mg). Be sure that some vitamin D is included with your calcium/magnesium supplement to help assimilation.

Yes, you will be taking a load of supplements every day and won't know if it all was worth it until you celebrate your 100th birthday and people ask you, "How did you do it?"

*The rationale behind taking relatively large doses of vitamin C is to mimic the quantities that would be made by the liver if we still had the ability to synthesize vitamin C.

3

CAUTION: THE AIR YOU BREATHE IS DANGEROUS TO YOUR HEALTH

The air you are breathing is killing you!

It's not from the cigarettes and cigars other people are smoking, and it's not from the cigarette in your mouth (even though that's a killer in itself), *IT'S FROM THE SMOG*!

What About SMOG? It Stings My Eyes A Little And Sometimes I Have To Cough A Little, But A Killer??

Okay, let's back off a bit.

We all know we must have oxygen to stay alive. Oxygen is necessary to combine with the foods we eat to give us the energy to run our body, rebuild cells and tissues, build new tissues, hormones, muscles, etc. The process is called oxidation.

However, even ordinary oxygen can be dangerous in certain forms which can attack and destroy normal cells. Certain overactive particles called FREE RADICALS are highly reactive and will combine with protein or other cellular matter changing the matter into material which can accelerate aging. Free radicals can be normal by-products of the body's metabolic processes and can be controlled, for the most part, by the body's defense systems.

The formula for oxygen is written 0_2.

But that's not the only formula containing oxygen. There's also 0_3.

0_3 is Ozone.

Ozone is one of the components of SMOG and is an oxidant.

Why Pick On Ozone? I Keep Reading In The Papers About The Ozone Layer And The Way It Protects Us From Solar Radiation.

When it stays up in the stratosphere it does protect us from radiation. It's like a fire in the stove. When it stays in the stove it provides warmth, light, and cooks our food, but, if the fire gets out into the middle of the room it can be a great danger.

The ozone in SMOG and the nitrogen oxides (also found in SMOG) have been listed by the World Health Organization as the two most important toxins worldwide.

SMOG, with its high concentrations of strong oxidants is a killer, responsible for more human disease and death than any other toxin or pollutant.

ON SMOG ALERT DAYS IN THE LOS ANGELES BASIN, FOR EXAMPLE, DEATHS IN NURSING HOMES SHOW A SHARP INCREASE!

SMOG affects all humans by increasing their susceptibility to respiratory disease and by decreasing the lung's ability to do its normal work.

SMOG can shorten your life!

And, it's not only in Los Angeles.

What About The Clean Air Act?

It's only an act and not an actuality. The Clean Air Act set a deadline that called for reducing ozone levels so that they do not exceed 0.12 ppm (parts per million) for any one hour period during any 24 hours.

According to the Environmental Protection Agency, *most* — if not all metropolitan areas in the USA did *not* meet the 1987 deadline and still have not cleaned the air to make it safer for human beings.

Where Does Ozone Come From?

Some ozone diffuses down from the ozone layer. Background levels of about 0.01 ppm are considered to be normal. But, much higher levels are formed when gasoline vapors and other hydrocarbons and nitrogen oxides mix with and react with sunlight and heat. The Los Angeles basin often is subjected to levels of ozone as high as 0.3 ppm.

That Doesn't Seem To Be A High Concentration. How High Does It Have To Go To Hurt Us?

Significant decreases in lung vital capacity in humans, that's you and I, are found for ozone levels as low as 0.3 ppm, and all pulmonary functions are affected adversely in humans who have breathed air with levels of ozone as low as 0.24 ppm.

Short term exposure to levels in excess of 0.5 ppm have caused acute changes in the respiratory function.

What Can I Do? I Have To Breathe And There's No Place To Move To.

Nature has a way of foreseeing the problems we make for ourselves and coming up with answers.

Our body can defend itself against oxidative stress by using antioxidant enzymes and nutrients. Back in the cave days when there wasn't the threat of gasoline and burning coal, early man was able to meet his body needs for antioxidants through the diet alone. He had to or you wouldn't be reading this today. Modern man, however, has difficulty in getting enough raw material to manufacture the defensive chemicals and usually has to resort to supplements.

The enzymes the body uses include superoxide dismutase (SOD), catalase, and glutathione peroxidase. The nutrients include vitamin E, vitamin C, vitamin A, beta-carotene, and the minerals selenium and zinc.

I Know That Vitamins Are Good For Us But How Are They Helpful Against SMOG?

SMOG makes us susceptible to infection, particularly pulmonary types of disease, and shortens the life span. Ozone and nitrogen dioxide (powerful oxidants) can cause pathological changes in a relatively short period of time unless they are neutralized. The protective nutrients sacrifice themselves to avoid damage to the cells.

How Do They Do That?

As stated previously, oxidants have one or more unpaired electrons. Electrons — when they are not paired — go crazy. It may be simplistic, but compare an unpaired electron to an animal in heat. An animal, so influenced, will mate with any other one of its species. The unpaired electron goes one step further — it will mate with any other electron it bumps into. The vitamins mentioned, particularly vitamin E, mate with the free radicals, thereby sparing the cells and tissues from damage.

Vitamins E and C are the most important antioxidant vitamins, athough vitamin A and its vegetable pre-form beta-carotene, are not far behind. Beta-carotene is actually two of the vitamin A molecules bound together. When the body needs vitamin A action, it uses an enzyme to cut the bonds and release usable vitamin A. This can be a better way to obtain vitamin A than from the usual animal sources such as from codfish because it is possible to overdose on animal vitamin A. It is not possible to overdose on beta-carotene since the body will not absorb it unless it is really needed. Diabetics should use fish liver oil since some diabetics lack the enzyme necessary to separate the A molecules.

Furthermore, animals given vitamin E live appreciably longer when exposed to ozone than do vitamin E-deficient animals.

(Fletcher, B.L. and Tappel, A.L. "Protective Effects of Dietary Tocopherol in Rats Exposed to Toxic Levels of Ozone and Nitrogen Dioxide". *Environmental Research.* 6: 165-175, 1973)

How Much Vitamin E Should I Take?

Vitamin E and vitamin C are among the least toxic of the vitamins. Vitamin E has been tested in humans at levels up to 55,000 International Units for five months and 3,000 I.U. for up to eleven years, and no side effects were reported. Except for some gastrointestinal disturbances in a few patients which were reversible, there is little evidence that doses of vitamin E up to any prudent amount is harmful.

In view of the low toxicity of vitamins and the potential benefit from defense against the oxidative damage of SMOG, it appears to be wise to take antioxidants as supplements.

Vitamin E in a dose of 400 I.U. and up to 1,000 milligrams of vitamin C should be a protective dose for at least some of the population. The other nutrients — selenium, vitamin A, beta-carotene, SOD, glutathione peroxidase, zinc — can be found in numerous combinations in health food stores and drug stores. Ask for a good antioxidant formula and read the label. It should contain, at least 400 IU of vitamin E, 10,000 IU vitamin A, 1,000 mg of vitamin C, 50 micrograms of selenium, 15 mg of zinc, and 15 mg of beta-carotene. If the formula also contains some SOD and glutathione peroxidase or catalase in any quantity, so much the better.

Follow the label directions. If there is a SMOG alert, double the dose for the time that the alert is in effect.

4

STRANGE NAMES AND STRANGE SUBSTANCES MAKE FOR A LONGER LIFE

Aspirin was a strange name at one time and so was Omega-3 fish oil, but we learned about them and found ways to use them in our search for a longer and better life.

Here are some more "strange" names. You'll begin to see more news about them as M.D.'s start to believe in their life-extending qualities and as more and more of the news media pick up on their unique abilities.

Germanium

Note: The FDA, in its infinite wisdom, has restricted shipments of germanium, as well as tryptophan. Although germanium is not available now, we feel it will soon be back on the shelves and that you should be aware of its potential benefits.

This is an example of what is called an ultra-trace mineral.

Less than fifty years ago many of the essential minerals were thought to be unimportant to human nutrition. Minerals like zinc, manganese, silicon, and chromium were ignored. Today, however, it is scientifically acceptable that all three are vitally important to proper metabolic functioning and to our total health.

Now scientists are studying a large number of other minerals, substances which are used by the body in ultra-trace amounts such as cobalt (which is part of the B^{12} molecule), silicon, gold, and germanium.

Isn't Germanium Something That Has To Do With Semi-conductors?

Yes. . . and so is silicon.

We do tend to confuse inorganic germanium with organic germanium. Inorganic germanium (a mined mineral) has been used as a semi-conductor (something that conducts electricity in an efficient manner). Inorganic germanium can be highly toxic even in small amounts.

Organic germanium (Bis-Beta-Carboxyl-ethyl Germanium Sesquioxide) has gone through considerable testing and has been found to be virtually non-toxic.

Organic germanium was only recognized as being potentially helpful to longevity about 30 years ago when a prominent Japanese chemist, Dr. Kazuhiko Asai became interested in it. He noticed that many traditional Chinese medicinal herbs contained germanium in high concentration.

How Does Inorganic Germanium In The Soil Become Organic "Safe" Germanium?

That's one of Nature's gifts. Somehow, the plants pick up inorganic material and turn it into organic material. They do the same for all of the essential minerals like zinc and iron. You couldn't eat iron ore or zinc metal and expect to get any nutritional benefits. You'd only get sick and perhaps even die. But once it has been through the plant it is now essential to health.

Many of our "healing" plants contain large amounts of germanium and some nutritionists think the power of those plants may be due to the high germanium content. You know some of those healing plants, such as ginseng, aloe, garlic, comfrey, watercress and chlorella.

Once Dr. Asai found that adding germanium to growing plants enhanced both growth and flowering, he decided to test germanium on animals. He found that it promoted the healing of serious wounds and even terminal disorders. Then, being a dedicated scientist, he decided to experiment on himself.

He had long been suffering from arthritis and rheumatism. Although the diseases were not life-threatening, they did interfere with his life enjoyment. Within a few weeks he noted a dramatic improvement in his condition and in his life appreciation. He talked about how he felt and people saw for themselves the improvement in his walking and general condition so the word soon spread like wildfire about his new "cure."

Many people with incurable illnesses asked to be treated with the new substance and soon Dr. Asai had enough material to write a book. He did so and related numerous case histories in, *Miracle Cure: Organic Germanium,* from which the following cases are cited.

Case Report:

A 24 year old female with cellular degeneration became unable to walk or write and even experienced difficulty in speaking. Taken from specialist to specialist, she was finally told there was no cure. After a month of treatment at Tokyo's Germanium Clinic, her speech impediment began to improve. After five months of treatment, she regained the ability to write and, in ten months, was walking again.

Case Report:

A 54 year old male was diagnosed as having cancer of the lungs. X-rays showed two malignancies in the right lung. Anticancer drugs had been used with no benefit; but after taking 500 milligrams of organic germanium a day for five weeks as nutritional therapy, he showed no trace of the malignancy.

These are accounts of clinical treatments done in Japan where a great deal of experimentation is taking place, and are part of worldwide evidence that germanium is remarkably effective in halting and reversing many disease processes *by restoring metabolic efficiency.*

How Does It Work?

There will have to be much more scientific investigation into germanium before that question can be answered exactly, but here's some of the answer.

It appears that the astounding cures of germanium result largely from its ability to "latch on to" three atoms of oxygen and bring them into the body.

It will be important to understand a little about the role oxygen plays in the body and how a deficit of oxygen can result in a shortened life.

Oxygen is the single most important element in human survival. We can live about one week without water and about a month or more without any food. But, if the body is deprived of oxygen for only a few minutes, cells die and we die as well.

Oxygen equals energy. We cannot run without energy. Energy moves our lungs, makes our hearts beat, removes poisonous wastes, keeps us young and alive! Severe oxygen deficiencies completely inhibit cell function, shutting them down and cutting off life. Milder oxygen deficiencies will impair the efficient functioning of the body's metabolism leading to eventual health decline. Once health is impaired there will be further reductions in body oxygen reserves and further illness.

For example, low stores of oxygen will result in the loosing of free radicals generated by ordinary metabolic processes. And an insufficient supply of oxygen means that more of the free radicals will escape and be able to enter and damage the reproductive capacity of cells and tissues. Also, those free radicals that are able to be trapped as they react with oxygen simply pull more of the body reserves out of action.

When oxygen stores are reduced the immune system is compromised, making it more difficult for the body to fight off disease. The presence of foreign invaders in the body calls for action by the white blood cells. White blood cells are the body's soldiers and they require increased supplies of oxygen to destroy invading bacteria and viruses. This need will further deplete oxygen stores, making replenishment for metabolic purposes more difficult.

Once the body is oxygen-deficient, certain pathogens can increase their growth. There are organisms that thrive in a low-oxygen environment. Candida is one such organism. Once it sets up a colony in the body, it begins to make the environment more suitable for its own comfort by manufacturing a substance called acetaldehyde (a bit like formaldehyde). This causes damage to the surrounding tissue and begins to use up whatever little oxygen there is left. Strangely, cancer cells have also been shown to prefer oxygen-free environments. Nobel Prize recipient, Otto Warburg, found that he could induce a cancerous transformation in vitro by reducing the oxygen concentration in cell cultures.

In summary, mild oxygen deficits will reduce the proper functioning of cells and pave the way for the development of chronic disease processes. The way to break the cycle appears to be to increase the oxygen stores in the cell.

Why Do We Become Oxygen Deficient?

The cave man didn't face an oxygen-deficient life. The oxygen in the air we breathe today has been greatly reduced by pollutants. That, plus the fact that we take in other pollutants through the food and the water we eat and drink, which must be detoxified through metabolic processes, increases the need for oxygen. Diets high in caffeine, alcohol and other processed or highly acidic foods predispose us to oxygen deficiency.

Acidity is recognized by the hydrogen ion. Hydrogen ions combine with oxygen to make water ($H^{2}0$). So, when there is a lot of acid in the body, oxygen is needed to neutralize the Hydrogen ions into stable water. Also, when we are under mental stress we secrete certain hormones such as adrenaline which tends to make the body more acid and once again contributes to using up oxygen reserves.

What Can Germanium Do Under Those Conditions?

Experimental studies have confirmed Dr. Asai's observations about the ability of this ultra-trace element to help replenish the body's stores of oxygen.

The three oxygen atoms attached to the germanium molecule act directly as an extra supply of oxygen and/or help the body to better use its own oxygen stores. Some experiments seem to be cruel even though they prove Dr. Asai's observations. In one such experiment, mice fed germanium were submerged in water. They survived much longer than a control group of mice who were not fed germanium. This demonstrated that the mice that had been supplemented with germanium had a greater amount of available oxygen.

Does Germanium Do Other Things To Help Longevity?

Experimental work has shown that germanium can stimulate the body's defense system against tumors. It appears to have interferon-inducing activity in both humans and animals.

Interferon works by inhibiting further cancer cell growth while stimulating the body's natural system of immunity. In a study using germanium it was noted that there was a normalization of T and B lymphocyte function (white blood cells which protect the body) and also stimulation of natural killer cells (NK cells) which run around the body killing suspected pathogens.

At the clinical level, germanium has been used with some effectiveness against a wide assortment of diseases including liver breakdown, high blood pressure, eye diseases, and a host of other malfunctions of the human body. The list of diseases which respond to germanium is so varied as to be almost unbelievable until one realizes that this is a natural substance. Unlike drugs which will affect just one particular enzyme or biochemical process, germanium works on the basic cell. It is for that reason that it can be effective in any condition that will respond to an improvement in the metabolic action of the basic cell.

Dr. Asai called germanium a health-giving substance because it restores health to those afflicted with disease, and sustains health in those who are healthy. He found that its effectiveness will be enhanced by eating foods low in acid such as fish and vegetables. For the same reason he said it would be wise to avoid mental stress and chemical pollutants whenever possible.

Is Germanium Harmful To The Body?

Tests have shown that organic germanium is non-toxic but, because it induces the excretion of toxins stored in the body, there may be a period of time when you feel a bit "out of it" when you begin to take it. This is because your body will get rid of life-long accumulations of toxins which will enable your cells to rejuvenate. But as they are excreted in the urine, feces, and through the pores of the skin, there can be a "healing crisis," an interim period, usually resolved within a period of two days to two weeks.

Suma (Pfaffia Paniculata)

While man is systematically destroying the rain forests in the Amazon basin to the detriment of the entire world, some men and women are trying to explore the native knowledge of herbal remedies in an effort to save and learn what other "primitive" cultures have learned through centuries of trial and error.

Though the surface of this priceless botanical resource has barely been scratched, many applications which may be of great use to mankind have been uncovered. One of them is the herb called Suma. It is a member of the Amaranth family, a cereal herb that is now being cultivated as a staple product for consumption in the United States. You've probably heard about Amaranth as a breakfast food and also as a substitute for rice or potatoes.

Suma is obtained from the roots of the Pfaffia Paniculata. The natives of the Matto Grosso in Brazil use it as a purifier, aphrodisiac, and for energy and healing. They call it "Para Todo" which means "for all things," symbolizing its varied use.

Modern herbalists place it in the category of adaptogens. Adaptogens appear to be natural substances which help us to adapt to new stresses and help restore natural immunity and immune resistance against stress. This restoration happens at the individual cell level and promotes regeneration and longevity.

Although it was known and used by the natives for over three centuries and classified in Europe in 1820, it was not studied until 1970 by Dr. Brazzazh, Chief of Pharmacology at the University of Sao Paulo. Samples were then sent to Japan to be researched for the reported health benefits.

The Japanese studied the herb and discovered a group of active constituents called pfaffosides, which are not found in any other plants. It is also strange that they have found strong concentrations of germanium along with the pfaffosides.

How Is It Being Used In The U.S.?

Although still under research and investigation, Suma is being used to increase and balance energy. One of the problems of aging is a decrease in energy and the desire to participate. Suma appears able to change that picture for the better.

Where Can I Get It?

Try your health food store and follow the label directions.

Speaking of Energy. . . Alpha-ketoglutarate

As we get older we feel the need for more energy, not only to exercise, but also to do the various tasks we have to just to keep ourselves from falling apart.

Pyridoxine (vitamin B^6) and a substance with the impossible name of alpha-ketoglutarate are essential elements in the body's production of energy. Since such production is critical to daily activity as well as keeping our body in shape for longer and better living, many substances have been examined as means of enhancing strength, stamina, endurance and speed of movement.

Aerobic activity is being cited as a means of improving our ability to ward off cardiovascular disease. Full aerobic activity is limited by a number of factors, including the circulatory delivery of oxygen to the muscles and the ability of the oxygen-burning engines in the cells (the mitochondria) to burn the oxygen as fuel in spite of the presence of waste materials such as lactic acid.

What Has This To Do With Increased Energy For Us?

It has to do with 1 + 1 = 3

No, there's nothing wrong with the mathematics, it's just that synergy and mathematical logic don't come out the same way all of the time.

When either pyridoxine and/or alpha-ketoglutarate are given alone, no significant effect on energy production is noted. However, when the two substances are bound together and given as one substance, there is a profound improvement in athletic performance.

That is the principle of synergy. Two substances that are unremarkable when taken separately into the body suddenly become different and stir the energy capacity of the body when bound together.

And that's not all!

The effect of binding vitamin B^6 to alpha-ketoglutarate can also be a promising event in the management of diabetes.

In one trial conducted by the Center for the Treatment of Diabetes and Metabolic Diseases, results showed that the combination of the two substances potentiated the effects of insulin and phenformin (an oral hypoglycemic agent) in lowering blood glucose concentrations while reducing blood lactate and pyruvate levels.

What's This Combination Called And Where Is It Sold?

It goes under various names including PAK but you'll have to ask at the counter of either health food stores or drug stores.

Follow label directions but do not use it for diabetes unless you ask your doctor about it first!!!

Silybum Marianum (Milk Thistle) and Your Liver

The liver is the most important organ of metabolism. It's known as the "chemical plant" of the body. The liver regulates fat, carbohydrate and protein metabolism, the storage of vitamins and minerals, and governs the detoxification reactions in the body.

Since the liver is the major site of detoxification of toxic chemicals, it is also at high risk for damage by such chemicals as DDT, dioxin, PCB's and other toxic compounds found in food, air and water. If you stop for one moment and think that the yearly production of synthetic pesticides alone is more than 1.4 billion pounds, then you have to be scared of the amounts we take into the body without our being aware of them.

Deaths due to liver damage are the fourth leading cause of deaths in the United States.

So, a longer and a happier healthy life can depend on how you help your liver.

Avoiding damaging chemicals is the first defense against liver damage. Also, avoiding self-pollution with alcohol and tobacco products is the next best defense. Then, next in line is a common herb called silybum marianum plus some other herbals in combination.

Silybum marianum is a member of the Compositae family. You know the family best by its more common member, the Daisy. silybum marianum can grow up to ten feet tall with large purple flowering heads. The plant is indigenous to both Western and Central Europe and is also found in the United States.

Here in this single plant, are several of the most potent liver-protecting substances known. The concentration of these substances is highest in the fruit of the plant.

Silymarin's effect of helping to prevent liver destruction occurs primarily from its ability to inhibit those factors that are responsible for the damage. Liver destruction occurs primarily as a result of certain toxins producing or acting as free radicals — highly reactive compounds that damage cells and tissues so that they produce distorted cells. Silymarin's components prevent that damage by acting as antioxidants. It appears that the antioxidant activity of silymarin is even more powerful than that of vitamin E.

Another way that the liver can be damaged is by the action of substances known as leukotrienes. These leukotrienes are compounds produced by the transfer of oxygen to a polyunsaturated fatty acid.

The action is produced because of the presence of an enzyme called lipoxygenase. Silymarin is able to inhibit the activity of this enzyme, thereby shutting down the formation of the damaging leukotrienes.

And, perhaps the most interesting effect of the herbal components on the liver is their ability to *stimulate protein synthesis*. The result is that *they actually build new liver cells to replace old, damaged cells.*

Perhaps the ravages of too much alcohol can be counteracted with this herbal compound and control of a drinking habit!

Experimental liver damage in laboratory animals, produced by such diverse toxicants as carbon tetrachloride and galactosamine, have been avoided when the animals have been treated with the herbal complex.

This combination has even been 100 percent effective against the severe liver poison of Amanita phalloides, the death cup toadstool/mushroom. Ingestion of this poisonous plant is about 30 percent lethal, but when the herbal compound was given to the animal before it ate the toadstool it was 100 percent effective in preventing any toxic effects.

Even if the herbs were taken ten minutes after the amanita toxin was ingested, they were able to counteract the toxic effects. If given within 24 hours, the herbs will prevent death and greatly reduce the liver damage.

What Can It Do For People Who Stay Out Of The Woods And Avoid Toadstools?

The only reason toadstools were mentioned is that their poison damages the liver so badly. However, there are a lot of people who are mushroom hunters and do make the mistake of not identifying the mushrooms correctly. If a doctor is not immediately available, this herbal compound can save lives.

In other human studies, silymarin has been shown to have dramatic results in treating several liver diseases, including cirrhosis and chronic hepatitis. The actions appear to be by preventing free radical damage to liver cells, by preventing the formation of leukotrienes and by stimulating the production of new liver cells.

What Are The Other Herbs In This Herbal Complex?

The others are extract of Cynara Scolymus (artichoke) and Curcuma Longa (curcumin).

The artichoke has a long folk history in treating liver diseases. Scientists have found that the active ingredient in artichoke is called cynarin and is found mostly in the leaves.

The cynara extract has demonstrated significant liver-protecting and regenerating effects. It also helps to promote the flow of bile from the liver to the gall bladder. This is protective because if the bile is not being adequately transported, there is an increased risk of damage. This action is very useful in the treatment of hepatitis and other liver disease via this "decongesting" effect.

Cynara typically lowers cholesterol in most cases because it helps to decrease the synthesis of cholesterol in the liver. Cynara extract has lowered both blood cholesterol and triglycerides in human and animal studies.

In a controlled trial, two groups of 30 patients having elevated serum cholesterol and triglycerides were given either cynarin 9500 mg a day) or a placebo. Cynarin proved to induce a significant reduction of the elevated cholesterol and triglyceride levels.

In addition, the patients also displayed a reduction in weight. This may have been due to cynarin's diuretic action.

The other herb, curcumin, is the yellow pigment of tumeric, a common kitchen herb. Curcumin shares some of the same effects on the liver as silymarin and cynarin.

Any Other Benefits From These Herbs?

Although this book primarily deals with life extending substances, the quality of the life must also be taken into consideration. Psoriasis, while not particularly life-threatening, does interfere with enjoyment of life.

There appears to be some connection between the use of silybum and some alleviation of psoriasis. Its efficacy is probably related to two factors: its improvement of liver function and its inhibition of the synthesis of inflammatory leukotrienes.

The link between the liver and psoriasis may be because of one of the liver's basic tasks, that is of filtering toxins from the blood. A functioning liver is able to filter out endotoxins which, if left circulating, make the skin condition worse.

A low-fiber diet is also associated with production of those endotoxins so a high fiber diet will also help psoriasis sufferers.

Of course, treatment of psoriasis should be under the direct supervision of a physician and the use of herbs can be in conjunction with other therapy. Usual dosage is one capsule three or four times a day. The herb can be purchased at health food stores and at some drug stores.

References to Silybum and Other Herbs

1. Regenstein, L.: *America the Poisoned.* Acropolis, Washington, D.C., 1982.
2. Wagner, H.: "Plant constituents with antihepatotoxic activity." In: *Natural Products as Medicinal Agents.* Beal, J.L. and Reinhard, E. (eds). Hippokrates-Verlag, Stuttgart, 1981.
3. Vogel, G., Tuchweber, B., Trost, W. and Mengs, U.: "Protection against Amanita phalloides intoxication in beagles." *Toxicology and Applied Pharmacology* 73:355-62, 1984.

4. Desplaces, A., Choppin, J., Vogel, G. and Trost, W.: "The effects of silymarin on experimental phalloidine poisoning." *Arzneim-Forsch* 25:89-96, 1975.
5. Hikino, H., Kiso, Y., Wagner, H., and Fiebig: "Antihepatotoxic actions of flavonolignans from Silybum marianum fruits." *Planta Medica* 50:248-50, 1984.
6. Vogel, G., Trost, W., Braatz, R., et al.: "Studies on pharmacodynamics, site and mechanism of action of silymarin, the antihepatotoxic principle from Silybum marianum." (L.) Gaert. *Arzeim-Forsch* 25:179-185, 1975.
7. Sarre, H.: "Experience in the treatment of chronic hepatotopathies with silymarin." *Arzneim-Forsch* 21:209-12, 1971.
8. Reynolds, J.E. (ed): Martindale: "The Extra Pharmacopoeia." *Pharmaceutical Press,* London, 1982.
9. Maros, T., Racz, G., Ktonaj, B. and Kovacs, V.: "The effects of Cynara scolymus extracts on the regeneration of the rat liver." *Arzneim-Forsch* 16:127-9, 1966 (1st communication) 18:884-6, 1968.
10. Vontini, M., Levoni, P., Angoro, A. and Pagani, G.: "Controlled trial of cynarin in the treatment of the hyperlipemic syndrome." *Arzneim-Forsch* 25:1311-4, 1975.
11. Pristautz, H.: "Cynarin in the modern treatment of hyperlipemias." *Wiener Medizinische Wocheschrift* 1223:705-9, 1975.
12. Kiso, Y., Suzuki, Y., Watanabe, N., et al.: "Antihepatotoxic principles of Curcuma longa rhizomes." *Planta Medica* 49:185-7, 1983.
13. Leung, A.: *Encyclopedia of Common Natural Ingredients in Food, Drugs, and Cosmetics,* John Wiley & Sons, New York, N.Y., 1980.
14. Rosenberg, E. and Belew, P.: "Microbial factors in psoriasis." *Archives of Dermatology* 118:1434-44, 1982.
15. Editorial: "Leukotrienes and other lipoxygenase products in the pathogenesis and therapy of psoriasis and other dermatosis." *Archives of Dermatology* 9:541-7, 1983.

The Ginkgo Biloba Tree

The Ginkgo is the world's oldest living tree dating back over two hundred million years. It has been called a "living fossil" having been able to survive the Ice Age but the species retreated to China and lived there until more recent times when it began to populate all corners of the world once again.

The Ginkgo tree has shown a remarkable resilience and resistance to insects, disease and pollution. For this reason Ginkgo trees are frequently planted along major boulevards and streets which carry heavy traffic and destroy more conventional trees. Individual trees may live as long as 1,000 years reaching a diameter of 3 to 4 feet. The tree bears an ivory-colored inner seed that looks like an almond. This seed is edible and is sold as a food in the Orient.

What Does This Have To Do With Life Extending?

The leaves of the tree were used as a dietary supplement by the Chinese, particularly the elderly, to promote longevity and resistance to aging.

Ginkgo's pharmacological activity is due to its high content of terpenes, flavonoids, pro-anthocyanidins and Ginkgo Heterosides (flavo-glycosides).

We Can't Eat The Leaves Even If We Had A Tree Growing In The Garden!

That's right. The leaves can collect pollutants on their surface that may be harmful, but there is an extract now available called Ginkgo Biloba Extract, or GBE for short. This extract has been made into tablets and can be purchased at your health food store.

The GBE is made from the leaves and has been shown to be active on different parts of the circulatory and nervous systems. Studies have shown the GBE to:

- Enhance intracellular energy production
- Increase cellular glucose uptake
- Inhibit platelet aggregation
- Demonstrate free radical scavenging activity
- Increase blood flow to the brain, and
- Improve the transmission of nerve signals

What Does All Of That Mean?

It means that the GBE can help people improve the way they feel in that they can be more energetic. It also means that the GBE can help make the blood more slippery so the chances of clotting in an artery will be reduced; that the GBE helps to fight free radicals, helps to make memory better and may even be of assistance in some cases of senility and Alzheimer's disease.

All this means a possible anti-aging extract from the world's oldest species of tree.

Where Can I Buy It?

Health food or drug stores will have it on their shelves. The usual dose is 40 milligrams three times a day, or follow label directions.

Latest on Ginkgo

In November 1992, *Lancet* published a review of *Ginkgo biloba* extract, summarizing the results of ten "well conducted, controlled trials." This is an excellent review article discussing the manufacture and nature of the European phytomedicine extracts used clinically for treating a variety of conditions. Of four different ginkgo preparations, only two have been used in controlled trials, one produced in Germany, and the other an Italian-made extract. These preparations are similar and are standardized to the same ingredients: ginkgo-flavone glycosides and terpenoids. *Lancet* refers to ginkgo as "among the most commonly prescribed drugs." Ginkgo is used to treat cerebral insufficiency, which includes twelve symptoms often experienced by the elderly:

Absentmindness	Difficulty of memory
Anxiety	Dizziness
Confusion	Headache
Decreased physical performance	Lack of energy
Depressive mood	Tinnitus
Difficulty of concentration	Tiredness

The article goes on to describe different studies, including randomized double-blind studies, documenting the effectiveness of ginkgo in increasing blood flow in the capillaries and decreasing blood clotting. Ginkgo extracts have been shown to improve metabolism in the brain and protect the brain against damage from oxygen deficiency. In two trails of elderly patients, both the German and Italian extracts caused a return to normal of the electroencephalogram in elderly patients with cerebral insufficiency.

This article also describes the prevention of membrane damage from free radical effects; that is, oxidative damage which is considered to be a part of the aging process.

Most importantly, after a review of all clinical research on Ginkgo biloba done to date, no serious side effects have been noted in any trial.

References:

1. Chatterjee, S.S. and Gabard, B. "Studies on the mechanism of action of an extract of Ginkgo Biloba, a drug for the treatment of ischemic vascular diseases." *Naunyn-Schmiederberg's Arch Pharnacol* 320:R52, 1982.
2. Beretz, A., Joly, M., Stoclet, J.C. and Anton, R. "Inhibition of 3',5' AMP phosphodiesterase by biflavonoids and xanthones." *Planta Medica* 36:193-5, 1979.
3. August, M. and Defeudis, F.V., Clostre, F. and Deghenghi, R. "Effects of an extract of Ginkgo Biloba on rabbit isolated aorta." *Gen. Pharmac.* 13:225:30, 1982.
4. August, M. and Clostre, F. "Effects of an extract of Ginkgo Biloba and diverse substances on the phasic and tonic components of the contraction of an isolated rabbit aorta." *Gen. Pharmac.* 14277-80, 1983.
5. Le Poncin, Lafitte, M., Rapin, J. and Rapin, J.R. "Effect of Gingko Biloba on changes induced by quantitative cerebral microembolization in rats." *Archs. Int. Pharmacodyn Ther.* 243-236-44, 1980.
6. Karcher, L., Zagerman, P. and Krieflstein, J. "Effect of an extract of Ginkgo Biloba on rat brain energy metabolism in hypoxia." *Naunyn-Schmiedeberg's Arch. Pharmacol* 327:31-5, 1984.

7. Vorberg, G. "Ginkgo Biloba Extract (GBE): A long-term study of chronic cerebral insufficiency in geriatric patients." *Clinical Trials Journal* 22:149-157, 1985.
8. Bauer, U. "Six-month double-blind randomized clinical trial of Ginkgo Biloba Extract versus placebo in two parallel groups in patients suffering from peripheral arterial insufficiency." *Arzneim-Forsch* 34-716-21, 1984.
9. Hindmarch, I. and Subhan, Z. "The psychopharmacological effects of Ginkgo Biloba Extract in normal healthy volunteers." *Int. Jrnl. Clin. Pharmacol Res.* 489-93, 1984.
10. Gebner, B., Voelp, A. and Klasser, M. "Study of the long-term action of a Ginkgo Biloba Extract on vigilance and mental performance as determined by means of quantitative pharmaco-EEG and psychometric measurements." *Arzneim-Forsch* 35:1459-65, 1985.
11. Schaffler, V.K. and Reeb, P.W. "Double-blind study of the hypoxia-protective effect of a standardized Ginkgo Biloba preparation after repeated administration in healthy volunteers." *Arzneim-Forsch* 35:1283-6, 1985.

The European Anti-Aging Complex — GH-3

In Germany, if a man or woman goes to the doctor complaining of prolonged depression, the doctor can prescribe something called GH-3 even though it can be bought over-the-counter without a prescription. After a few days most patients claim that the blackness has "lifted."

In Mexico they can get injections of Gerovital if they feel that age has "dragged them down."

In Switzerland, cell injections plus procaine can revive old feelings, including those involved with sexual pursuits.

In Romania, routine injections of GH-3 increase overall well-being and sharpen minds.

But, in the United States, GH-3 is only legal in the state of Nevada and sometimes by mail from Life Extension, Inc., P.O. Box 2276, Boca Raton, Fla. 33427-2276.

What Is This GH-3?

GH-3 or Gerovital therapy began in Rumania in 1946 when Dr. Ana Aslan, now director of the National Institute of Gerontology and Geriatrics in Bucharest, began using it to treat various disorders associated with aging. In September, 1956 she spoke before an international symposium on aging and said that Gerovital could do the following:

- regenerate the body at the cellular level
- eliminate depression
- increase energy, vigor, and overall vitality
- normalize high blood pressure
- improve libido and sexual potency
- alleviate the pain and stiffness of arthritis
- relieve chest pains
- improve the memory
- alleviate the symptoms of senile brain disorders
- restore youthful skin texture and appearance

Sounds Like A Miracle... Is It?

Consider this: it is used in more than 45 government-sponsored clinics in Rumania, as well as other clinics throughout Europe and most of the world. Only the U.S. does not allow it to be sold, except for two instances.

As a matter of fact, a form of Gerovital called procaine or Novocaine is used as a local anesthetic to ease the pain of dental work. Gerovital also contains benzoic acid and potassium metabisulfite and elements to lower the acidity of the procaine solution. This combination makes the drug penetrate biological tissue and fluids more readily and makes it able to reach its target areas in a potent form. Whereas conventional procaine breaks down into para-aminobenzoic acid (PABA — one of the B-vitamins) and diethylaminoethanol before it reaches the brain, the procaine in GH-3 appears to be able to reach the brain in its original, potent form.

The diethylaminoethanol (DEAE) is known in medicine as a blood pressure regulating substance so if a little is produced from the GH-3 it just helps to regulate pressure.

Dr. Aslan refers to her mixture as a "vitaminic factor" but the FDA and the Merck Index refer to it as a prescription drug which makes it unavailable to the general public from health food stores.

Has There Been Other Research Work Done To Prove Or Disprove GH-3?

There was a British research team headed by a Dr. Robinson. They found that there was a strong connection between relatively high levels of an enzyme called oxidase (MAO) in the blood serum and the brain, and the overall aging process.

Other researchers at the University of Southern California — Professor J.P. Hrachovec, for example — demonstrated that procaine is able to inhibit MAO. It is interesting to note that high levels of MAO have been associated with depression and that MAO inhibitors have been used with eye-opening success in the treatment of that depression.

When the circulatory system ages, the whole body ages. Decreases in mental capacity and memory have been linked to arteriosclerosis or hardening of the arteries. According to a Dr. E. Pakesch of Vienna, disturbances in the mental performance have evaporated with procaine therapy.

Dr. R. Baker observed that blood cells lose their flexibility and get more rigid as they age. When treated with procaine they don't get rigid as fast as they would without it.

A Dr. B. Zuckerman, working with laboratory nematodes, demonstrated that aging can be delayed with procaine.

Is Procaine Something New?

No, it's been around since 1905 when a doctor Alfred Einhorn wanted to find a synthetic substitute for cocaine. That's the reason the two names are so much alike. Dr. Einhorn combined two naturally occurring substances, PABA and DEAE and came up with procaine. Unlike cocaine, procaine is not psychologically addictive and the body does not build up a tolerance to it to require progressively larger doses.

Throughout the time it has been used in dentistry it has been shown to be an excellent local anaesthetic, but it also has other beneficial qualities. It can stimulate the blood vessels to widen, permitting easier blood flow, relax the muscles, calm down an overactive thyroid, and reduce the severity of allergic reactions.

How Come Nobody Noticed Its Revitalizing Action?

No one injected procaine and then observed the subjects over a long period of time. It wasn't thought of as a revitalizing substance, just as a pain killer!

Then, in the forties, Dr. Aslan began using procaine on arthritics at a government clinic. She injected it into the painful joints, which relieved the pain as expected, but there was also the unexpected result that her patients appeared to be getting younger. The texture of their skin improved, their memories sharpened, their vitality and muscle strength increased.

These results encouraged Dr. Aslan to test procaine further. One of the tests involved 15,000 people and was so successful that the government set up the 144 clinics in various areas of the country.

People talk about its revitalizing power, but doctors want more testing done before it is legally recognized and approved for use. According to the tests done so far, Gerovital is quite safe and effective.

You also have to understand that Rumania was a socialist country and authorities were not as interested in keeping people young as they were in keeping people productive! The trials of GH-3 were mainly to see if this substance could help the aging worker do a better job for the state. Obviously the officials were satisfied that there was an increase in capacity and productivity or they wouldn't have opened so many clinics.

Antidepression and Revitalization

If we examine the relationship between depression and revitalization, the way some U.S. doctors limit their approach to GH-3, we find the following list of symptoms:

- depressed mood characterized by sadness and despondency
- hopelessness and gloom

- an inability to experience pleasure
- poor appetite and weight loss
- insomnia or too much sleep
- loss of energy and fatigue
- agitation
- decrease in libido
- loss of interest in work and other activities
- self-reproach or guilt
- loss of ability to concentrate
- confusion
- loss of memory
- sense of helplessness and hopelessness
- anxiety or tension
- physical complaints, real or imagined

Wow! It's quite a list of symptoms.

To a lot of people it may sound like what happens when you grow old. In truth it is the FDA's official list of guidelines for defining a state of depression.

But consider that our skin and tissues also become "depressed." And our attitudes become "depressed." Aging is in the mind as well as in the body.

According to some theories, our body was designed to be immortal.

It protects itself against poisons and infectious diseases.

It heals itself when it is injured.

It is an effective machine when given enough raw material to keep itself in balance.

But, for as yet unexplained reasons, it loses its balance and body systems lose their ability to self-maintain. . . and we age!

Aging is not only on a biochemical basis but on a psychological level as well.

A happy, vigorous state of mind will support and stimulate a vital HEALTHY BODY!

Gerovital helps revitalize us by maintaining a homeostatic balance in the critical areas of the brain. This translates into maintaining a balance between all the brain chemicals which are responsible for many important functions, including mood, energy, sexual potency and so on. Those chemicals are called neurotransmitters and they control all the communication that goes on in the brain. They're how the brain talks to itself.

The key neurotransmitters are serotonin and noradrenaline. When people are healthy, these substances coexist in the brain with little problem. But that balance is threatened by another chemical, monoamine oxidase or MAO. MAO is an enzyme that is able to break down noradrenaline. If there is too much MAO present in the brain, the balance is disturbed and there is an excess of serotonin. This causes depression and fatigue!

Usually, MAO is not present in the brain in excess amounts but *as we age, MAO levels in the brain begin to rise*. Usually the buildup begins in earnest around the ages 40 to 45.

Boy! All We Have To Do Is Take Something That Knocks Off The MAO!

It's not that easy. We did make a lot of drugs to do just that but they all had similar problems. Not only did they destroy MAO in the brain, but also in the rest of the body as well. Elsewhere, it turns out, MAO has some important function, like helping to regulate blood pressure, and is necessary for certain vital liver functions. So, it can't just be turned off all over.

So What Does GH-3 Do?

It appears that Gerovital is a "weak inhibitor" of MAO, meaning that it can help to control MAO in the brain but doesn't interfere with its actions when it is needed elsewhere in the body.

Why Can't We Get It Everywhere In The U.S.?

Maybe politics plays a part. The FDA has not approved it and, because it cannot be patented, drug companies are not interested. Also, the most effective way to take it is by injection. There are tablets of GH-3 but absorption from the stomach is not as easy. Of course, tablets are better than not having GH-3 at all.

References:

1. Schwarzhaupt. Cologne, Germany.
2. G. Bruening. *Aerztliche Praxis*, 22, 4064, 1970.
3. H. Marx. *Fortschritte der Medizin*, 79, 299, 1961.
4. H. Suttinger. *Aerztliche Praxis*, 20, 1491, 1968.
5. Meeting. "Theoretical Aspects of Aging." Miami University, Miami, FL, 1972.
6. E. Robinson, et al. *Lancet*, 5, 290, 1972.
7. J.P. Hrachovec. *Fed. Proc.*, 31, 604, 1972.
8. J.P. Hrachovec. 26th Annual Meeting of the Gerontological Society, 1973, Miami Beach, FL.
9. E. Pakesch. *Wiener Klinische Wochenschrift*, No. 82, 211, 1970
10. J. Weiss, H. Glazer, L. Poherecky. *Psychology Today*, No. 8, 58-60, 1974.
11. S. Cohen, K. Ditman. *Psychosomatics*, No. 15-19, 1974.
12. D. MacFarlane, H. Besbris. *Journal of the American Geriatrics Society*, No. 8, 365-71, 1974.
13. A. Mock. *Aerztliche Praxis*, No. 22, 1999, 1970.
14. A. Gelenberg, et al. *Am. J. Psych.* 137, 622-623, 1980.
15. B. Zuckerman. 26th Annual Meeting of the Gerontological Society, Miami Beach, FL, Nov. 1973.
16. J. Officer. 26th Annual Meeting of the Gerontological Society.
17. R. Baker. 26th Annual Meeting of the Gerontological Society.

Things Go Better With CoQ

The CoQ in this case is the substance called Coenzyme Q-10.

Your body cannot make Coenzyme Q-10, but you cannot survive without it.

If your body supply of CoQ drops 30 percent below your normal amount, numerous degenerative process begin and organ after organ in your body grows old.

Where Does It Come From?

We get it from our food.

But, according to the research done by Dr. Karl Folkers at the University of Texas, and by Dr. Emile Bliznakov at the New England Research Institute in Connecticut, the ability of the liver to convert the CoQ found in food into the CoQ-10 (the only form found in humans) *declines with age.*

Healthy Longevity

Recent evidence suggests that deficiency is a strong possibility and that CoQ-10 supplementation has a place in a sensible anti-aging program.

For example, Bliznakov gave 50 aging mice weekly injections of CoQ and compared them with 50 mice of the same age which did not receive any CoQ-10.

The CoQ mice remained vigorous and healthy.

The control group declined, became inactive, and died of old age!

After nine months the last of the control group was dead but 20 of the CoQ group were still alive and active.

Three of the mice lived 38 months, a lifespan equivalent to a human life of 145 years.

How Does CoQ Have Such An Anti-aging Effect?

We'll explore some of the virtues of CoQ as we go on, but one clue lies in the immune system. Evidence of the effect of CoQ in being able to stimulate the immune system has been accumulating since early in the seventies. It appears that CoQ-10 is able to increase the activity of the white blood cells, the protective body cells that seek out and destroy invading bacteria and viruses.

When there is a decline in CoQ, as there is with aging, there also appears to be a decline in the immune function. If there is less immune action, the body is less able to deal with invading bacteria and viruses and therefore there is more disease and more wear and tear on the body.

But, in experiments done by Folkers, older mice who had lost most of their immune function were given a single injection of CoQ. They regained their capacity to produce antibodies — a measure of immune strength — almost to the level of young mice!

(Folkers, K. and Wolaniuk, A. *Drugs Under Experimental and Clinical Research,* 1985, 11, 539-546.)

But there's more!

The immune stimulating effect of CoQ-10 may even be strong enough to fight cancer. Bliznakov and his staff induced cancer in mice by injecting them with a potent carcinogen (cancer-causing agent) called dibenzopyrene which is the most potent agent in cigarettes. One group of injected mice was also given CoQ and the rest were left untreated.

At the end of ten weeks, every one of the untreated mice had developed tumors. Twenty-five percent of the treated mice never developed tumors throughout the study.

(Bliznakov, E. *Biomedical and Clinical Aspects of Coenzyme Q,* Elsevier Biomedical Press, N.Y. 1977, 77-83.)

So, one way to retard aging is to maintain a strong immune system by using supplements that assist that purpose.

CoQ-10 and Heart Disease

Study into CoQ began in 1957 when a scientist, F.L. Crane, and his research team, first extracted it from animal tissue. Their initial research concluded that CoQ was able to remove or add oxygen to or from important body molecules. This is important because a lack of oxygen can produce a fall in cellular energy but too much oxygen can result in the formation of toxic free radicals.

The highest concentration of CoQ in the human body is in the heart muscle. Some researchers think that one of the major factors in heart disease is the decline of CoQ in heart tissue as we age.

Cardiac patients have significantly lower levels of CoQ throughout the body than healthy people and most cardiac patients show CoQ deficiencies in the heart muscle.

In 1982, Mortensen and his group at University Hospital in Copenhagen, showed that the severity of myocardial infarction (heart attack) is directly correlated with the degree of CoQ-10 deficiency. The most severe cases had about half of the CoQ-10 level of healthy hearts.

(Mortensen, et al, *Drugs Under Experimental and Clinical Research,* 1985,11)

Nobuyoshi, et al confirmed these findings of severe CoQ-10 deficiencies in heart patients at Kokura Memorial Hospital in Kitakyushu, Japan. Then those patients received 90 milligrams of oral CoQ-10 daily for two weeks. The heart and blood levels of CoQ-10 increased for those patients.

(Nobuyoshi, et al, *Biomedical and Clinical Aspects of Coenzyme Q*, Vol. 4. Elsevier Science Publishers, New York, 1984, 221-229.)

Japan is the leader in the use of CoQ-10. It is reported that nearly 6 million Japanese now use this substance each year, primarily for mild congestive heart failure and other disorders. In numerous clinical studies, over 70 percent of the patients treated with oral CoQ-10 showed clear beneficial results.

It may be that one of the anti-aging effects of CoQ-10 may stem from its action in protecting the heart from a CoQ deficiency.

Is It Possible To Explain How CoQ Works Without Getting Too Complicated?

Each cell has a tiny motor to produce power for the cells to operate. The motor is called the mitochondria. CoQ-10 plays a critical role in pumping protons across the mitochondrial membrane, and without this action the body would not have enough energy to stay alive.

CoQ-10 serves the same function as the cylinders in an automobile engine where the gasoline is ignited and explodes to drive the piston. Without CoQ-10 the cell is like a dead engine: there is no spark or ignition.

Where Can I Get This?

If you want to use it as a supplement, most health food stores and drug stores have it. It comes in many strengths but the usual dose is 10 milligrams three times a day.

For medical use in various illnesses such as heart problems or dental problems you should consult your doctor or dentist.

What Does It Do For Dental Problems?

In 1975, experiments showed that CoQ was effective in reversing gum disease. This is important because about 40 percent of Americans have chronic gum disease and as many as 32 million will lose teeth because of it.

Dr. E.G. Wilkinson, an Air Force Dentist, pioneered research into CoQ and gum disease. He and his team took samples from dental patients with periodontal disease and found that they showed a marked deficiency of CoQ. Supplements were able to stop the progress of the disease and initiated extraordinary healing of gum tissue.

According to Dr. Wilkinson, periodontal tissues are deficient in CoQ when they are diseased and appear to require more CoQ to heal.

Recent research has shown that periodontal disease is not just limited to gums but is a generalized disease with a heavy involvement of the immune system.

Another reason for the success of CoQ treatment of gum disorders is the proven ability to stimulate an immune response.

There are other benefits to supplementation with CoQ-10. Sedentary people, even "couch potatoes," can improve the heart's performance and strength without having to exercise. It means that supplementation may be a good idea for the person who doesn't want to follow a regular program of exercise. It doesn't mean that you can take it and then run a marathon. Just that you will be able to get heart support.

Blood pressure has been lowered simply by adding CoQ-10 to the diet. No medication was used in a study that lowered the pressure from 141/97 to 126/90 after two months.

It is obvious that CoQ-10 supplementation might extend life in some cases because of its effect on heart health and on the immune system during a diseased state.

Another aspect of aging is antioxidant capacity. CoQ-10 is able to normalize oxidation by adding or removing oxygen from vital tissues.

Overweight people may have a CoQ-10 deficiency condition. When CoQ-10 was given during a controlled study, the group who took CoQ-10 and a set diet lost 29.7 pounds compared to the control group which lost 12.7 pounds. In other words, it makes your diet lose twice as much weight for you as it ordinarily would. And you lose fat so fast, there's no time for you to binge and break the diet.

What Foods Naturally Contain CoQ?

Meats, mackerel and sardines. Bran cereals, peanuts, spinach and broccoli. But the problem may be the conversion of natural CoQ to CoQ-10.

References:

1. Bliznakov, E.G., et al. "Coenzyme Q: stimulants of the phagocytic activity in rats and immune response in mice." *Experientia* 266:953, 1970.
2. Folkers, K. and Y. Yamura, eds. *Biomedical and Clinical Aspects of Coenzyme Q.* Vol. 2. Amsterdam: Elsevier/North Holland Biomedical Press, 1980, pp. 333-347.
3. Judy, W.V., et al. "Coenzyme Q-10 reduction of adriamycin cardiotoxicity." Folkers and Yamura, Vol. 4, 1984.
4. Kamikawa, T., et al. "Effects of coenzyme Q-10 on exercise tolerance in chronic stable angina pectoris." *Am. J. Cardiol.* 56:247, 1985.
5. Kishi, T., et al. "Bioenergetics in clinical medicine. XI. Studies on coenzyme Q-10 and diabetes mellitus." *J. Med.* 7:307, 1976.
6. Mayer, P., et al. "Differential effects of ubiquinone Q-7 and ubiquinone analogs on macrophage activation and experimental infections in granulocytopenic mice." *Infection* 8:256, 1980.
7. Oda, T. and K. Hamamoto. "Effect of coenzyme Q-10 on the stress-induced decrease of cardiac performance in pediatric patients with mitral valve prolapse." *Jpn. Cir. J.* 48:1387, 1984.
8. Shigeta, Y., et al. "Effect of coenzyme Q-7 treatment on blood sugar and ketone bodies of diabetics." *J. Vitaminol.* 12:293, 1966.
9. Suzuki, H., et al. "Cardiac performance and coenzyme Q-10 in thyroid disorders." *Endocrinol.* Japan. 31-755, 1984.
10. Vanfrachem, J.H.P. and K. Folkers. *Coenzyme Q-10 and Clinical Aspects of Coenzyme 9.* Amsterdam: Biomedical Press, 1981.

11. Van Gaal, L., et al. "Exploratory study of coenzyme Q-10 in obesity." Folkers and Yamura, Vol. 4, 1984, pp 369-373.
12. Wilkinson, E.G., et al. "Bioenergetics in clinical medicine. II. Adjunctive treatment with coenzyme Q in periodontal therapy." *Commun. Chem. Pathol. Pharmacol.* 12:111, 1975.
13. Yamagami, T., et al. "Reduction by coenzyme Q-10 of hypertension induced by deoxycorticosterone and saline in rats." *Internat. J. Vit. Nutr. Res.* 44:487, 1974.

More Energy Aids — Bee Pollen

What's old is new again. The Council on Alternative Medicine has authorized a study of bee pollen as a means of controlling allergies, but it has always been highly regarded for its energizing properties. Because of its wealth of nutrients, bee pollen has been prized for its effectiveness in combatting fatigue.

It seems that this unique supplement is rediscovered every few years. In the January 25, 1977 issue of the Philadelphia Enquirer, the great sprinter Steve Riddick is quoted as saying that bee pollen helped him to anchor the United States 400-meter relay team and to win a gold medal at the summer games in the Montreal Olympics. He said he had popped three bee pollen pills each morning before breakfast for three years.

He said the pills made him run easier and faster and that his recovery time after a hard sprint was quicker. Pollen also helped him build his stamina.

Before Steve Riddick, the famed distance runner from Finland, Lasse Viren, trained on bee pollen in the sixties. After using bee pollen, he won the 5,000- and 10,000-meter Olympic races. And former Russian Olympic track coach Remi Korchemny, who has moved to the United States, has experimented with bee pollen for years.

One of the major frustrations of the human mechanism is the aging of the body and skin. That, along with a loss of energy, is symbolic of advancing years. Bee pollen, with 185 nutritional ingredients and 22 amino acids, can help your skin become clear and firm, and help the furrows and wrinkes become less conspicuous. Although bee pollen does not have the effect of plastic surgery, the changes that occur are extremely beneficial to the skin.

At your health food store. Follow label instructions.

More Energy Aids — Inosine

It began when the Japanese were searching for a substitute for digitalis. Digitalis is a drug used by heart patients, most of them elderly, suffering from an irregular heartbeat or from angina. Digitalis acts to promote continued smooth cardiac operation.

So does Inosine, but there's more.

Inosine belongs to the chemical family known as purine nucleotides. It is able to penetrate the cell wall of muscles of the skeletal type and of the cardiac type. Once inside it helps to promote the production of ATP.

ATP (adenosine triphosphate) is the fuel used by the mitochondria (tiny engines inside each cell) to make energy.

It also promotes the production of another biochemical called 2,3 diphosphoglycerate (2,3, DPG). This biochemical is essential for facilitating the transport of oxygen from the red blood cells to the cell's engine for energy.

So, what inosine does is move oxygen into the cell to help burn the ATP it has helped to manufacture. The result is more available energy to help you move better, feel better, exercise better or have sex better. Without energy you feel old!

The Japanese have touted their discovery as helpful in the treatment of heart problems and, when prescribed in medical doses, it probably is. However, when athletes discovered inosine they found that they could do away with the harmful anabolic steroids because inosine helped them in the same way but without the harmful side effects.

Unless you suffer from gout, excess uric acid in the blood which causes pain and swelling in the joints, inosine appears to be free of any noticeable ill effects for otherwise healthy individuals.

You can get it in health food and drug stores and follow label directions.

You Say Inosine Can Offer The Same Results As Harmful Steroids. What Can Steroids Do And Where's The Harm?

Fair question.

It's no secret that bodybuilding changes your muscles. Not only does it make you stronger but it also makes your muscles much larger.

The bodybuilding effort is good for your bones because it exerts pressure on them, stresses them and makes them stronger and less likely to be prone to osteoporosis.

Strenuous exercise also eats up body fat and cholesterol and improves your immune system.

So far so good!

You look better. . . up to a point, have stronger bones and muscles and find that you can resist disease more easily than the next guy, unless he's a bodybuilder as well.

Muscles grow when they're stressed in a correct manner and shrink when they are no longer stressed on a regular basis.

Muscles grow proportionally larger when they are stressed and you take anabolic steroids at the same time.

Muscle becomes stronger via bodybuilding through two basic mechanisms:

Stress exercise builds better fiber motor unit recruitment through nerves. You use more muscles and you use them more efficiently.

Muscle also becomes stronger through individual fiber hypertrophy. Exercise stress increases the cross-section diameter of each muscle fiber. As individual muscle fibers hypertrophy and/or increase in number, the muscle enlarges.

When you exercise, the contractions of the muscle induces the muscle cell to draw protein into itself. So it grows!

Each person has a built-in genetic capability to build muscle. Once you build a muscle you must exercise it to keep it large and strong.

Where do anabolic steroids appear in this scenario?

Steroids are drugs.

Steroids alter the receptor chemistry of muscle cells.

In essence, steroids command the DNA in the nucleus to make more cell protein. When the muscle is stressed in the presence of steroids it will grow larger than without the steroids.

NOW, BEFORE YOU RUN OUT AND TRY TO BUY STEROIDS, LOOK AT WHAT YOU HAVE TO LOSE. . .

Your liver has to detoxify the steroid and muscle residues in the body. This detoxification process is the same as detoxifying poisons. Eventually, the liver cells can't take it anymore and either grow cysts or quit altogether.

Vascular areas can form into tumors.

Your immune system is threatened.

You can come down with arthritis, bursitis, asthma, allergies, muscle inflammation, heart attack, atrophy of the testicles, etc.

Not a pretty thought or a pretty set of symptoms!

That's why steroids are forbidden in the Olympics.

The better route is nutrition, using vitamins, minerals, bee pollen, octacosanol, glandulars, amino acids and. . . inosine.

Steroids are killers, not at once but somewhere down the road. Avoid them like the plague!

Cytochrome C — The Fatigue Fighter

We've devoted a lot of space to energy and fatigue because people lack these elements and that lack contributes to the cycle of growing and acting older. Energy makes people feel younger and exercise make the body look and feel younger.

Cytochrome C is a simple chemical compound that is produced in the body naturally. It is composed of a number of amino acids plus iron. This compound acts as a carrier of oxygen within the mitochondria in each cell. It is also a part of the complex process that allows your muscles to do work.

According to the latest scientific research, the amount of cytochrome C in the muscle will skyrocket the length of time your muscle will perform before it runs out of fuel and fatigue sets in. That means before the muscle burns and cramps and you have to sit down or stop whatever you are doing.

Even if you're not in shape, your performance can be improved by the addition of cytochrome to your daily diet.

Whenever you exercise, even when you do nothing more than walk a few miles, the various metabolic processes of your body need oxygen. If your body does not have enough cytochrome C it will switch over to another method of obtaining energy termed anaerobic (without oxygen).

This anaerobic method produces lactic acid buildup which causes your muscles to burn and cramp. You may even feel the pain the next day or so. This lack of cytochrome C could explain why some people tire so easily no matter how little they do.

By supplementing your diet with cytochrome C you can raise your exercise tolerance levels without boring or vigorous training.

This exciting fact should lead many of you to include a couple of cytochrome C tablets with breakfast to go all day. Get them at the health food or drug store and follow the label.

Pau d'Arco, Taheebo, Lapacho Morado, Ipe Roxo

All of these names apply to a legendary herb from a tree of the botanical family Bignoniacea, tecoma, conspocua. It is one of the tribal remedies of the Callawaya Indians of South America.

South American physicians are using this Indian medicine, inherited from the ancient Inca Empire, to treat various life-shortening diseases.

A brew or tea made from the inner bark of lapacho colorado appears to attack the cause of the disease, particularly when it is of the debilitating type.

Lapacho Colorado, or red lapacho — so called because of its scarlet flowers — grows in the warmer part of South America: Brazil, Northern Argentina, Paraguay and Bolivia. It was also in common pharmacopoeia of the native tribes called the Tupi-Nambo Indians and the Guarani long before the advent of the Spanish in the New World.

The tree was called by different names but used for similar ailments in the various areas in which it grows. Ipes is the name used in southern Brazil so the tree is named Ipe Roxo. Some tribes used the wood of the tree to make their bows for archery so their name is Pau d'Arco or "bow stick."

The introduction of this medicine to Western civilization is romantically tied up to a more-or-less modern legend. About 30 years ago at Americans, a suburb of Sao Paulo, Brazil populated by descendants of the Confederacy who homesteaded the land at the invitation of Emperor Dom Pedro II after the South was lost, a young girl was stricken with a virulent form of cancer.

The medical establishment had given up on the girl and told her parents that she didn't have long to live. But an aunt contacted the local medicine man, an Indian herbal doctor, who said that he could help the girl with a tea made from the bark of a tree which grew in the area.

At first, the suggestion was treated with the disdain most moderns have for herbal medicine, but then the girl had strange dreams. She saw a priest who urged her to drink the tea brewed from the bark the Indian had given to her. As the pain increased and the dream was repeated, she decided to try the tea.

The pain slowly diminished and she continued to drink the brew. After a time, so the story continues, she was found to be free of disease.

At the celebration party, one of the guests was a medical doctor from the town of Santo Andre who took a sample of the bark for his own study. His brother was also stricken with the same disease. The condition was "inoperable and terminal." The doctor, Dr. Orlando dei Santi, went directly to the Municipal Hospital of Santo Andre where he was a resident physician. He took the bark, boiled it in white wine, mixed the still hot juice with orange juice and let his brother drink it on an empty stomach. After a month of this "unorthodox" treatment, the brother was able to leave the hospital and go home.

After this startling treatment became known in the hospital, many physicians began breaking the rules of established medical investigation, which call for testing and testing substances before they can be tried on human subjects, and began to use the bark for a variety of diseases. Since 1960 it is a standard treatment at the hospital and many herb stores and pharmacies stock the bark for their customers.

There have been scientific studies conducted on this botanical for a number of years by Dr. Theodoro Meyer, recipient of the Argentine National Prize for Biological Sciences, and Professor of Botany and Plant Geography of the National University of Tucuman. He isolated the element xyloidin as an antibiotic with virus-killing capabilities. An elixir (liquid concentrate) made from three specific species of the Bignoniaceas is prepared and distributed throughout Argentina.

While examination of the herb hasn't presented conclusive evidence regarding its curative abilities, another element has been isolated and identified. It's called lapachol. Xyloidin and lapachol are the main elements in treating tumors and fungi. Other investigations say that it is an effective analgesic sedative, decongestant, diuretic and hypotensive. Because of its anti-viral capability it is also said to be active against any cold or flu virus.

So What... I'm Not Going To Go To South America!

You don't have to. The herb, usually in the form of a powder that can be used to make tea, is now available in the United States at most health food stores. No claims are made for it. There can be some uncomfortable side effects since some people have gotten diarrhea after drinking too much and, because it is a plant, some people may be allergic to it. On the whole though, it is a safe tea. It may be a life-extending herb or merely a refreshing brew depending on who you talk to.

Chinese Herbs

Life extension Chinese style is concerned with two basic objectives. Removal of the cause of illness by restoring balance and harmony to the body, and reinforcement and revitalization of the body's natural defense system.

Naturally, herbs figure into this life extension plan. A fully functioning immune system is in the forefront of defense against the elements which would cut short our lives. Our immune system is constantly on guard and we'll talk more about it later on in this book.

Many herbal books are to be found in libraries and on the shelves of book stores and health food stores, so I will not go into the whole listing of herbs but instead concentrate on some of the not-so-familiar herbs that the Chinese use to enhance the immune response.

Astragalus

This herb has been shown to double the survival rates for cancer patients undergoing chemotherapy or radiotherapy. It also is able to normalize many body functions and is effective against the common cold.

Codonopsis

Nearly identical in power to ginseng, this herb has been used in the treatment of heart palpitations, menstrual disorders and breast cancer. It stimulates red blood production, not white blood cell production, but it does enhance the transformation of white blood cells into the more effective T-Cells.

Schizandra

This is a stimulant herb with the ability to affect the central nervous system of healthy people. It is an energy tonic that enhances mental function. It also relieves insomnia. Chinese doctors often prescribe it for infections of the lungs and the gastrointestinal tract.

White Atractykodes

This substance is used to reduce platelet aggregation in the treatment of cardiovascular disease.

Ligustrum

Degenerative disorders such as chronic backache, loss of hearing or premature graying of the hair respond to this herbal.

Ganoderma

This substance is derived from the mushroom called rei-shi. It is now being cultivated in California although it was previously found only in the Orient. It enhances the immune system and has been used in the treatment of viral hepatitis where it has helped 70 percent of the cases.

Can a Mossy Tea Help Alzheimer's?

The caveman didn't have to worry about high blood pressure, arthritis or Alzheimer's disease.

He didn't live long enough!

However, the Ancient Chinese worried about their aged parents memory loss and, in their scientific approach to the problem, began experimenting with herbs and other natural substances. When they discovered a means of improving memory, it became part of their materia medica.

For hundreds of years, a tea brewed from a primitive form of life — a club moss — had the power to "perk up" people's memories.

As usual, Western medicine turned up its collective nose at the notion that the moss (*Huperzia serrata*) could have any effect on memory.

But, 7 years ago, researchers at the Shanghai Institute isolated a compound from that lowly moss that is "a potent inhibitor of acetylcholinesterase."

That discovery made all the difference in the world because acetylcholine is one of the most important chemical messengers in the brain and it is deeply involved in memory and awareness!

Wow! Isn't That What Alzheimer's Is All About?

Xu-Chang He, a chemist at the Institute, explained that acetylcholinesterase breaks down acetylcholine so it can't carry messages any longer. However, if the tea stopped the breakdown of the chemical, the messages could continue clear and loud.

When the news reached the Mayo Clinic in Jacksonvlile, Florida, the moss ingredient, now called huperzine A, became the object of an intense research campaign to see if it could be used as an agent against Alzheimer's disease which affects memory and afflicts over 4 million Americans.

According to Alan P. Kozikowski, a chemist with the Mayo Clinic, huperzine A is more effective and more specific than the prescription drug Tacrine, currently being used for the disease.

However, it's a long way from Florida, through the FDA, into drugstores.

Why Can't We Buy Some Dried Club Moss, Make Tea, And Use It The Way The Chinese Have Done For Centuries?

Maybe, by the time this book is published, you'll be able to get teabags of it at your local health food store.

Just when I finished writing about the Chinese herb for Alzheimer's, another article relating to the same herb and some others, came across my desk. This one in the *Journal of Ethnopharmacology*, 1993; 38(2-3), 129-135. "Plants in treating senile dementias in the northeast Amazon." Richard Schultes. The author has spent 50 years researching the plants used for medicinal purposes in the northern Amazon and remarks about the Indians of the area and their respect for the aged. At least 25 plants are used for Alzheimer's disease or similar problems. The plant leaves or roots are made into tea and used over a period of several days or even months. The following may or may not have the same inhibiting affect on acetylcholinesterase, but seem known for their palliative effects on the elderly:

- *Justica ideopgenes*, a member of the Acanthus family is used to treat palsley-like trembling.
- *Unonopsis veneficiorum* from the Custard Apple family is mixed with food for people who have forgotten how to talk.
- *Uonopsis stipitata* also helps the elderly with speech problems.
- *Tabernaemontana heterophylla* is in use when old people are slow and forgetful.
- *Pagea recurva* of the Gential family is used to treat debilitating forgetfulness.
- *Gnetum nodiflorum* is used for elderly men who cannot walk straight and totter or fall.

Along with the forementioned *Huperzia serrata, Galanthus nivalis*, an herb that contains the alkaloid galanthamine (another acetylcholinesterase inhibitor), is used to improve memory in the aged.

It's amazing that these "primitive" cultures have devoted so much energy and time and actually discovered substances that help their aged population while the vaunted medical associations seem to have so few resources at their fingertips.

And Then There's Anti-Aging Plants From China

What could be better than the contribution of plants to both the well-being of the aged and the prolongation of their lifespan?

Once again, we turn to the *Journal of Ethnopharmacology*, 1993; 38 (2-3): 167-75. "Immunological aspects of Chinese plants as anti-aging drugs," Xiao, Pei-Gen, et al.

From 365 plants described as "able to improve the vital energy of the body and maintain youth," the author has chosen 5 plants.

(Note: In order to insure that the correct plant can be found — when it is available in Western stores — the botanical name is used as an introduction. While it may seem cumbersome to read, it serves to differentiate plants which may sound alike but have different properties.)

- *Herba epimedii, Epimedium sagittatum, E. pubescens* is used to replenish vital functions especially sleeping sexual nerves.
- *Fructus Lycii* is prepared from the dried fruit of *Lycium barbarum*. It is a favorite ingredient in the treatment of the elderly. It also has been shown to improve sexual disorders in elderly animals. In humans, it decreases hyperlipidemia and senility symptoms.
- *Radix Plygoni Multiflorum* prolongs the life cycle of somatic cells, increases cellular antioxidant activity, lowers the waste material that accumulates in heart tissue, inhibits the formation of oxidized fats. . . and lengthens the lifespan of Japanese quails.
- *American Ginseng* shows the same protective ability and is also recommended by the author.

NOTE: Not all health food stores carry Chinese herbs so you will have to ask around in order to find them. Usually they are in combination with other herbs, all designed to work together in the Chinese manner to heal and to prolong life.

If you can't find Chinese herbs locally you might want to write to: The Institute of Traditional Medicine, 2017 S.E. Hawthorne, Portland, Oregon 97214.

More About Adaptogens, Schizandra and Acantho Root

In the 1970's, the Soviet Academy of Sciences in Vladivostok began a search for the truth about certain of the plants known by reputation to be healers. They were plants that grew in Tibet, North Korea and Siberia. They sent out teams of researchers to gather any plants which had been used by herbal healers for long periods of time and then subjected them to testing to find out if their healing properties were factual or fable.

The researchers gathered some 350 different plant species for testing and by the time they were through only a few were labeled as being healing plants.

Three of the researchers, Professors Brechman, Dardymor, and Lebedev, told the academy that a few of the plants tested were startling in their abilities, with properties that appeared to go beyond that of the vitamins and minerals they possessed.

They said the plants contained a "new" nutrient that possessed healing powers not found in any other comparable substance.

Once this was told, new research was initiated to find out how this "new" nutrient could be isolated. Research was not limited to the Soviet Union. Here, in the United States, Dr. Norman Farnsworth, chairman of the Department of Pharmacology at the University of Chicago, began his own studies. The plants under consideration were found to contain the "new" nutrient, confirming the studies done in Russia.

Other European countries, particularly Sweden under the direction of Karl-Otto Aly, M.D. of the Swedish Herbal Institute in Goteborg, began the investigation of the new nutrient and its relationship to health and longevity.

It was at that time that a name was needed instead of just calling it "new." The scientists decided on the name, "adaptogen," because it is a vital substance that reportedly helps people enjoy a longer and more active lifestyle.

Adaptogens appear to be biologically active substances similar to vitamins and minerals but, unlike these nutrients, adaptogens are found in only a few plants.

Although they can be used in the same way as other supplements, they appear to be able to offer protection from, as well as healing for, many ailments. Adaptogens may be the "fountain of health."

Researchers say that the use of adaptogens may bring these immediate benefits to the user:

- an improvement in energy production and distribution during periods of stress, whether mental or physical
- stimulation of the body's defense system to provide greater resistance to disease
- quicker recovery from respiratory diseases
- increased vim and vigor
- increased stamina
- increased strength
- protection against radiation

It also appears that adaptogens can help to reduce elevated sugar levels in the blood and exert a normalizing effect on blood pressure. They are also able to relieve general tiredness and increase mental alertness. But, perhaps the most interesting effect is their ability to help the body shield itself against infection.

Not all plants contain adaptogens. In fact, only two particular plants found in the regions tested were considered to be a "powerhouse" of adaptogens. And, the combination of the two was found to be even better than either of them alone.

The Soviet researchers identified the two as Schizandra chinensis, and Acanthopanax senticosus (simply called acantho root). They are powerful when used alone but the combination appears to be even better.

Schizandra had a reputation for healing way back in ancient days when it was included in the *Yellow Emperor's Study of Inner Medicine,* by Pen-tsao in 2700 B.C. In that ancient work it is credited with the ability to increase energy, replenish the internal abdominal organs, improve vision, boost muscular activity, and be helpful to colds and digestive upsets.

Once the adaptogens from schizandra had been isolated, the Russians found that they could aid the central nervous system, intensify mental and physical activity, enhance cardiovascular tone, improve a sluggish respiratory tract, and stabilize blood pressure. All of these qualities are important to longevity.

It is strange that adaptogens do not have a specific effect on an individual organ or process in the body directly. Instead they act via basic and regulating processes.

In other words, they help the body help itself to health. They, somehow, correct the disorder — whatever it may be — by instructing the body to unleash its own self-regenerating power.

While all nutrients are valuable and required for life, only these adaptogens appear to be able to stimulate the self-revitalization ability inherent in every cell but weakened due to sluggishness and old age.

The other half of the combination, acantho root, is able to increase physical strength and lengthen life expectancy. As reported in the *Swedish Pharmaceutical Journal,* No. 7, 1978, acantho root has a normalizing effect on many body processes. It is able to balance body functions. It is a detoxifier, boosts recovery after surgery, and helps in cardiovascular malfunctions.

When schizandra and acantho root are taken together, along with some other herbs to help carry them throughout the body, they are the most efficient adaptogens known to date. The Swedish Institute pointed out the following results:

- anti-stress reaction
- increased energy supply
- increased the production of proteins and nucleic acids
- helped in rheumatic heart disorders
- helped in diabetes
- aided gastric ulcers
- normalized blood pressure
- created an effective, overall robust feeling

These combinations are available at most health food stores and at some drug stores.

Follow label directions.

Echinacea

Miracle drugs cost millions to develop but nature has developed a number of miracle herbs and offers them to us at a fraction of the cost of the "laboratory miracles."

For centuries, this herb has been used by common folk against infections and inflammations. They didn't know anything about its chemistry but they did know that it worked. Now, modern science has finally taken a long look at the herb and has come up with explanations for its success in treating those and other conditions which affect longer life.

Its primary action is on the immune system, regulating the balance of antibodies to counteract the growth of unfavorable bacteria and viruses. It appears that these dangerous enemies spread by releasing the enzyme hyaluronidase which weakens the cell walls and makes it easier for them to penetrate into the cells and either destroy them or make them turn out more dangerous substances.

Echinacea can inhibit the production of hyaluronidase, the "spreading factor." Some studies shown in German research have shown that the body's overall immune response is increased by the herb's stimulation of the white blood cells called T-Cells which are able to attack, digest and remove pathogenic bacteria and viruses as well as their chemical toxins.

Echinacea is available in health food stores and in some drug stores. It can be purchased in liquid or tablet form. Follow label directions. It is particularly helpful during the colds season.

(Wang, C. *Advances in Chinese Medical Materials Research,* 1985, p.519-527. "Immune-Enhancing Effects of Ginseng.")

Two saponins and a polysaccharide have been found to stimulate the production of white blood cells in normal mice and in mice which have tumors. The ginseng promoted the production of antibodies when administered either by injection or when given orally.

(Atal, J. et al. *Journal of Ethnopharmacology*, 1986, 18, p. 133-141, "Immunomodulating Agents.")

An herb, picrorhiza kurroa, has been tested as a stimulant to both cell-mediated and humoral immunity and found to be very active. This has significant medical applications since immune system activity and long life are related.

Diabetes Shortens Life

But an herbal remedy used in Mexico can help to control it.

A type of cactus used in Mexico as an herbal remedy for non-insulin-dependent diabetes actually does lower patient's blood glucose levels.

According to an article in *Diabetes Care*, January 1988, the scientists who observed the results are still unclear as to why the cactus works.

After fasting for a 12 hour period, one group of subjects was given broiled stems of the cactus, opuntia streptacantha, which is used as a food in Mexico. Another group was given plain water. The blood glucose levels of the group taking the cactus decreased but the group taking plain water showed no difference.

It is possible, said Alberto C. Frati-Munari and his colleagues at the Hospital de Especialidades in Co. a Rasa, that the cactus improves the effectiveness of available insulin which stimulates the move of glucose from the bloodstream into the body's cells where it can be used as energy or stored as fat.

(*Science News*, January 23, 1988, p.62)

We Know That Stress Shortens Life

Do you know why?

When you are stressed — angry, anxious, hostile — your body releases hormones.

Those hormones were needed when we lived in caves 50,000 years ago and had to run or fight to survive.

But now, when most threats are not life-threatening, the body doesn't know it and still reacts as though a cave bear was considering you for a snack!

The hormones released are adrenalin and noradrenalin and, if they're not used up in a hurry, they tend to increase plaque in the arteries.

Cortisol is released from the inner part of the adrenal glands which diminishes the activity of the immune system! And, if you don't cope well with the situation, your DNA repair system gets depressed, among other things.

What A Mess, And Your Own Body Caused It.

It's hard to avoid stress but, like my old grandmother used to tell me when I got too upset over a trivial thing, don't pay a dollar for a penny's worth of trouble!

She also told me about some herbs which help in the calming-down phase.

Make a mixture of:

1 ounce of St. Johns wort
1 ounce of Lavender
1 ounce of Lemon balm

Use one teaspoon of the mixture to a cup of boiling water.

Remove from the heat and let steep for 3 minutes.

Strain, add honey to taste and sip slowly.

The Vitamin That Isn't — B15

The Russians think that B15 has near miraculous properties but the Food and Drug Administration in the United States doesn't want it to be sold.

B15 is chemically N, N-Dimethylglycine (DMG). It is not a vitamin because there is no convincing evidence that it is *essential* to human nutrition. For any substance to be considered a vitamin it must meet certain criteria. Its lack must cause a deficiency disease that can be recognized, the way that a lack of vitamin C causes the condition known as scurvy.

When B15 was isolated some 35 years ago by Dr. E.T. Krebs, he called it vitamin B15 because it is found along with other members of the B-complex family of vitamins. Like the B-complex vitamins, it is non-toxic and water soluble, with a vitamin-like chemical structure that resembles the vitamin PABA or choline.

What Does This Substance Do For You?

That depends on who you ask.

According to the research done in Russia, DMG does the following:

- Extends cell life
- Improves blood oxygenation
- Stimulates the immune response
- Plays a role in energy transport
- Plays a role in protein synthesis
- Helps protect the liver from pollutants
- Speeds recovery from fatigue
- Helps to regulate the level of steroids in the blood
- Helps to detoxify body pollutants

For example, brains grow old because their oxygen flow slows down. DMG forces those 40-plus brains to breathe deeper.

It's like you lit a fire under your mental powers. You think quicker and deeper. You remember more, and recall memories faster.

Many diseases have been treated in Russia with the help of DMG. The following list must be examined critically since we do not know what other treatment was used along with the B^{15}.

- Aging
- Alcoholism
- Allergies
- Cirrhosis
- Dermatitis
- Diabetes
- Drug addiction
- Heart disease
- Hepatitis
- Hypertension
- Neuralgia
- Neuritis
- Sciatica
- Senility

How Does It Work?

Basically it does three things: stimulates a more efficient use of oxygen by the body, nullifies some body pollutants and improves fat use.

Tissue respiration, the taking in of oxygen and the giving off of waste material, has been improved with DMG. When the cells respire with efficiency, less oxygen is required for their operation. This would make it helpful in the treatment of respiratory diseases including asthma and emphysema.

Increased tissue respiration is also effective at the brain level. This can be a factor in mental retardation. It also may account for some of the reports about its ability to afford relief from hangovers. Besides this, when used for alcohol addiction it appears to help the patient resist the craving for a drink. (Might be a good companion to the stated use of L-glutamine, an amino acid that has been used to help alcoholics lose their addiction.)

The ability of DMG to help in oxygen shortness, such as hypoxia, has caused some researchers to speculate about its possible value in the treatment of certain cancers.

Pollutants in the blood from food, air, water or even from some of the foods we eat, as well as some pollutants we manufacture in the body during normal metabolism, all compete with our body cells for the oxygen that is carried in the bloodstream. DMG has the ability to detoxify these pollutants through a process called *methylation*.

When these pollutants are methylated, they consume less of the available oxygen, making more of it available for cellular function which can benefit people who have narrowed arteries. DMG also helps to maintain cellular health to prevent premature aging, it helps aging athletes compete and gives younger athletes increased vigor.

An article in the *National Enquirer* states that the increase of oxygen at the tissue level accounts for its success as an energizer. When DMG is used, the effects can be felt within an hour and can last up to fifteen hours.

DMG appears to also lower the lactic acid content of the blood after muscular activity. This helps to reduce muscle fatigue and the burning sensation so many of us get after exercising. The burning and cramps can usually be felt the next day as well when DMG is not taken so it appears to work longer than could be expected. Long distance runners taking DMG were amazed at the increase in endurance. Some of them say that they were able to increase their endurance by as much as 25 percent. They felt better and recovered faster than ever before.

DMG and the Heart

Heart disease and related ailments cut short more American lives than all of the other death causes lumped together, according to the American Heart Association. Diet appears to be the main reason that 20th century man is in such poor condition. One reason may be a lack of natural sources of DMG, since DMG participates in fat dispersal, tissue respiration and detoxification.

The Russians consider DMG to be one of the prime supplements, to be used mainly for support of other cardiovascular disease treatments. When used with patients whose disease was associated with deficiency of the oxidative metabolism, a positive effect was noted with 80 to 90 percent of all patients treated. There was a disappearance of labored breathing and a general feeling of increased well-being. And, there was a note in the research which indicated that a combination of DMG and vitamins A and E was even better than DMG alone.

Because we are a culture that derives a good portion of its calories from processed foods, the first such culture in history, we are not getting natural DMG because it does not exist in foods that have been so processed. Some sources of DMG are brewer's yeast, raw seeds, whole grains that are unprocessed, and brown rice.

DMG and Free Radicals

Finally, the Russians say it holds back the erosion of time by burning up the poisons that rip apart our bodies at the cellular level, sending reinforcements against "free radicals," the nasty high-energy fragments that can hasten old age. According to Professor Yakov Shpirt, DMG is a potent stimulant in the control of aging.

And now for the Bad News

Here's where I usually tell you where you can get DMG.

Even though it is a virtually non-toxic substance with no side effects, the FDA doesn't want to hear about it.

Only one company has a DMG product on the market and it's hard to find.

But There's Also Good News — TMG

I wouldn't go through all of this to tell you about a supplement to help ward off aging and then leave you with a negative thought.

DMG is not easily found but TMG is readily available at health food stores and some drug stores.

TMG is trimethylglycine and may even be better than the original. TMG breaks down in the body into DMG plus extra methyl groups for the methylation process.

TMG does everything that DMG does and so effectively that athletes are using it for increased energy and recovery in all sports.

It's available as TMG or sometimes called free-base betaine. Don't confuse it with betaine hydrochloride which is a completely different supplement used to increase the hydrochloric acid content of the stomach when there are digestive difficulties.

TMG can be found alone or in combination with other vitamins.

As usual, follow label instructions.

Carnitine: The Fat Converter That Works From Within

Fat in the body, whether on your hips or roaming the bloodstream, can be a deterrent to a longer life.

Carnitine plays an important role in converting that roaming fat into useful energy because it transfers fatty acids within the cell to the energy-producing engine where the acids can be burned away. So, it takes the free-floating fat in your bloodstream and burns it for fuel.

Because carnitine can be manufactured in the liver, from the amino acids lysine and methionine, it is not considered to be an essential nurient. But, although our bodies can make it provided there is enough nutrient support, we obtain most of it from our diet, specifically from the darker organ and muscle meats.

However, because so many of us have cut down on meat-eating and rely more on vegetables, there is a greater chance of carnitine deficiency. Also, as we age, the mechanism for the manufacture of carnitine becomes less efficient and may result in a shortage of this substance. So, if you've cut down on meat and still haven't lost weight, then you need carnitine to finish the streamlining job you've begun.

As a fat converter, carnitine has been shown to be of benefit to people with cardiovascular problems on one end of the scale and for athletes at the other end. It is said to be useful for people with cardiovascular problems because it assists in regulating fat metabolism in heart and skeletal muscles. Some of the shown benefits include reduction of blood triglycerides and cholesterol, improvement of heart muscle exercise tolerance, prevention of irregular heartbeats, and an increase of energy for the heart.

Carnitine is also used by people with obesity problems because excess fat can shorten life. According to Dr. Jeffrey Bland, senior research associate at the Linus Pauling Institute of Science, carnitine plays an important role in the control of a condition called ketosis. Ketosis is believed to be the result of a loss of important minerals like potassium and magnesium. The loss affects the coronary system and causes an imbalance in electrolytes.

Carnitine helps to increase the efficiency of fat metabolism. People with diabetes or on a weight-loss program are more susceptible to ketosis because there is a decrease in fat metabolism.

A lack of carnitine can result in several disorders. Obesity can occur because of a fat build-up. Hypoglycemia can also occur and, if unchecked, can result in progressive muscular weakness, muscle disorders, heart tissue damage, an increase in triglycerides, a breakdown in muscle tissue, and irregular muscle function.

For athletes, carnitine supplementation produces more efficient fat burning which is necessary during prolonged strenuous exercise. It is even more important when you consider that the level of fat utilization for muscle energy rises as much as 60 percent during the heavy exercise period. Carnitine is also said to increase exercise time, prevent muscle fatigue, increase oxygen uptake, maintain normal energy metabolism and increase stress tolerance.

Most of those findings stem from animal research. However, recent research on carnitine has involved human athletes, to test the endurance factor.

Is It Useful For Both Men And Women?

Studies have found a considerable difference in the level of need for carnitine between men and women, with men having higher blood concentrations of carnitine. High levels of carnitine are found in the epididymis of the testes in men and adequate levels of it are found to be necessary for energy metabolism within the sperm for proper motility and fertility.

So it's fair to say that, although both sexes must have carnitine in sufficient amounts, men may need more for fertility.

Current Therapeutic Research, 30:753, 1981

Kosolcharoen and colleagues demonstrated significantly improved tolerance to exercise in patients suffering from coronary artery disease with L-carnitine.

American Journal of Cardiology, 43:300, 1979

Thomsen and colleagues proved increased tolerance to exercise when L-carnitine was administered to patients with coronary artery disease.

International Journal of Tissue Reactions, 11:175, 1980

Double blind study of patients suffering from angina pectoris. The group receiving L-carnitine showed noticeable improvement.

Lancet, 1:805, 1978

L-carnitine can significantly reduce total blood lipids (fats and fatlike substances).

Johns Hopkins Medical Journal, 150:51, 1982

1 gram of L-carnitine taken daily over a period of ten to fifteen weeks produced a substantial increase in high density lipoprotein (HDL) the "good" cholesterol, the cholesterol that is *protective* against coronary artery diseases.

Medical Hypotheses, 8:269, 1982

McCarty suggests that L-carnitine may be a useful supplement for those on a low-calorie diet. He hypothesizes that L-carnitine, by enhancing the efficiency of fatty acid oxidation (increasing the burn rate of calories stored as fat), may make low calorie diets easier to tolerate by reducing feelings of hunger and weakness that result from less efficient oxidation of fats.

Precaution

L-carnitine is a natural substance but there is another substance called D-L carnitine that is not recommended for use. Make sure that the substance you buy as a supplement says L-carnitine on the label and follow the label directions.

Do not use L-carnitine to treat an illness unless you are so advised by a physician who is familiar with the use of this substance.

Antioxidants and Free Radical Stress— Secrets of Prolonged Life and Prolonged Youth

Oxygen is the Dr. Jekyl–Mr. Hyde substance in our search for prolonged life and youth.

Picture this. . . on one side is the life-giving value of the oxygen we draw into our lungs.

On the other is the oxygen which attacks and corrodes body cells and steals life a bit at a time.

It's called aging, and yes, it can be slowed down!

Until recently the idea that we could actually extend life and continue to look younger and younger than previous generations had was considered to be only a dream, but that was before nutrition became more of a science. Now, scientists believe that they have discovered a means of controlling some of the aging process by the use of antioxidants. According to Dr. Benjamin S. Frank, M.D., aging is now a treatable disease.

Dr. Denham Harman, M.D., University of Nebraska

Today it seems very likely that the assumption that there is a basic cause of aging is correct and that the sum of the deleterious free radical reactions going on continuously throughout the cells and tissues is the aging process, or a major contribution to it.

Dr. Lawrence Badgley, M.D.

Until recently, the medical sciences lacked a unified theory of how disease occurs in the body. Well, this has all changed. Now there is the *Free Radical Theory of Disease* and it has a lot of support from many different branches of science and medicine. Whenever a group of scientists from different fields can generally agree on a theory, you may be tempted to consider that the theory is close to the truth.

Stephen Levine, Ph.D. and Parris M. Kidd, Ph.D.

The major enzymes defending against free radicals in the cell are superoxide dismutase, glutathione peroxidase and catalase.

(The above statements were taken from Baranowski's booklet, "Free Radicals Stress and Antioxidant Enzymes," 1987.)

The human body is composed of billions upon billions of individual cells acting together to form a cohesive unit called a person, me or you. Each cell, at the appropriate time, splits to form two new cells. If we could insure that each new cell was an exact duplicate of the "mother" cell we wouldn't show any signs of aging. The process of splitting is called replication or mitosis.

But, that's where the problem begins. Each subsequent cell is a little bit different from its parent. That's the result of stress, toxins, poisons, diet, environment, and *oxygen*.

And the older a cell becomes, the more susceptible it is to damage from free radicals.

What really prevents cells from copying themselves exactly? Researchers confirm that our bodies deteriorate and degenerate because cells are constantly under attack by corrosive, oxidizing molecules. Of course, all of us are exposed to stress — chemical, emotional, physical, and the stress that comes from infections. Chemical stress can come from pesticides, insecticides, heavy metals, asbestos, polluted air and water and radioactive wastes. When we think of all of the stresses we have to bear it's a wonder any of us stay healthy.

What Is A Free Radical?

A free radical is defined as any molecule which has an unpaired electron in its outer orbit.

We've all seen pictures of molecules. There's the center, like the sun, with electrons spinning around it like the planets. Each of the molecules in our body has that arrangement, with the electrons spinning around *in pairs*. The fact that they are in pairs keeps the molecule in balance. If, for any reason, the molecule loses an electron from its outermost ring it becomes *unbalanced*. It goes crazy, becomes unstable and begins to commit hostile acts against the body. It will rape, pillage, or steal an electron from any cell it can in an effort to become balanced itself.

We could applaud its effort to balance itself except for the fact that the cell it steals an electron from will now itself be damaged and will reproduce a less-than-perfect replica of itself.

When there is an excess of free radical activity in the body, we are destroying more cells than we can create. With cell death we have tissue death. With tissue death we have organ death.

Where Do They Come From?

In general, the stresses of living.

But, they are also manufactured in the body during normal cellular metabolism.

All day long we have to create energy to keep our body functioning. We combine food nutrients with oxygen to make ATP (adenosine triphosphate, the basic fuel of the cell). As a by-product of this normal operation some free radicals are formed. These particular molecules are oxygen molecules with an unpaired electron. Because of the unpaired electron, the molecule is now called *superoxide*.

Some Important Antioxidant Enzymes

SOD

Under normal conditions, these radicals are kept in check by an enzyme which is an antioxidant. Its name is superoxide dismutase (SOD) for short.

But, when we are exposed to stress, any kind of stress, the PRODUCTION OF THESE FREE RADICALS TENDS TO INCREASE AND EVEN REACT WITH OTHER MOLECULES TO FORM EVEN MORE TOXIC RADICALS.

The most common free radical generated from an excess of superoxide molecules is the *hydroxyl.* It's made when a superoxide mates with hydrogen peroxide.

The three most dangerous specimens are superoxide, the hydroxyl, and hydrogen peroxide. They are on the "ten most wanted list" in the body. They are the most common by-products of metabolism and are most responsible for cell damage.

The antioxidant enzymes manufactured by the body are our most important protection against these age-inducing molecules. . . that is, *as long as we can manufacture them in the quantities necessary.*

How Did All This Get Started In The Beginning?

When the Earth was young, the atmosphere contained gasses but there was no oxygen.

Then, as plant life began to evolve, a complicated balance began. Plants give off oxygen and take in carbon dioxide. As the rest of life evolved, it did so in an oxygen rich atmosphere. Plants found that the oxygen they got rid of was destructive to them and evolved mechanisms to protect themselves, so it's no surprise to find that most antioxidants used in supplementary form are obtained from plants.

Certain nutrients found in the plants we eat as foods can contribute to antioxidant protection. Briefly mentioned here, they will be the focus of attention later on.

The most important are:

Vitamin C	Bioflavonoids	Selenium
Vitamin B^6	PABA	Zinc
Vitamin E	Folic Acid	Magnesium
Vitamin B^3	Pantothenic Acid	Vitamin A

However, because there is such a large group of substances contributing to the formation of free radicals, it is questionable that even the best of diets can supply them in sufficient amounts.

When the free radicals attack, they can turn natural fats in the body into *rancid fats*. That's called lipid peroxidation. It is a major factor in aging and disease because all of our cells are surrounded by cell membranes and composed in part of fatty tissue.

When cell membranes become rancid, they are either hardened so that nutrients needed for nourishment cannot enter the cell, or the wall is punctured so that the cell collapses as the fluid slowly drains out.

We are all familiar with the process known as wrinkling. The skin cells collapse and harden, the skin sags and looks a lot like that old leather jacket you have hanging in the closet.

Another aging effect of free radical activity is inflammation, commonly called arthritis. There is a lubricant within the joints, put there by nature to help the joints move freely and without friction and pain. It's called synovial fluid. When this fluid is attacked by free radicals, it loses its lubricating quality and the joint becomes inflamed and unable to function with the ease of youth.

Although these are only two of the devastating actions, free radicals may be at the root of most of our aging problems.

How Do Antioxidants Help Us?

The superoxide dismutase removes the superoxide molecule, the glutathione peroxidase scavenges the peroxides and also hydrogen peroxide, and methionine reductase removes the hydroxyl radical while catalase also works on hydrogen peroxide.

If We Don't Make Enough Naturally, Can We Take Supplements?

That depends on who you listen to!

Supplementation with antioxidants was a controversial issue in the past because orthodox medicine didn't even believe in using vitamins therapeutically, much less antioxidants to help us live longer. This was especially true in the case of SOD.

SOD was first isolated in the early fifties but it was not until the 80's that the media began to acquaint people with its possibilities. It was the media which began to tell people about its antiaging claims. That was not so far-fetched because SOD does remove the most common free radical found in man, the superoxide radical.

Because of the publicity, a number of companies put SOD tablets on the market without sufficient study into how it works in the body and how to get it into circulation. The first tablets never made it into the bloodstream because the stomach acids simply ate them up. The people who took the tablets weren't getting the results they had read about in the papers and magazines.

So, the researchers went back to the drawing board and decided to coat the tablets with a substance that would protect it on its journey through the stomach to the small intestine. This was called an "enteric coating," and worked just as the researchers thought.

But, there is another problem. How much SOD is needed to be effective?

You and I manufacture about 5,000,000 units of SOD and its helper catalase each day. If we take 5,000 units and expect it to work we're only fooling ourselves. It's like taking vitamin C. If we take 10 mg. the body doesn't even notice it. We have to take vitamin C in the 100's or thousands. It's that way with SOD. We have to take a large enough dose to be able to liquidate the free radicals and 5,000 units is just not enough.

Glutathione Peroxidase

Also, SOD is never found alone. It's accompanied by friends, mostly by catalase and another of the body's major antiaging substance and free radical fighter — glutathione peroxidase.

Glutathione is made up of the amino acid glutathione and the important trace mineral selenium. When there is a team up of these two substances they can combat the free radicals specifically called *peroxides*.

According to Dwight Kalita, Ph.D., research director for the Huxley Institute of Biosocial Research of Ohio and his collaborator, research scientist Steve Blechman, this is a list of glutathione's functions:

- it is an antioxidant and deactivator of free radicals
- it it is a detoxifier of heavy metals and drugs
- it is an aid in the treatment of liver and blood disorders

- it plays an important role in the aging process and immune systems
- it is an aid in the treatment of allergies, hypoglycemia and arthritis
- it is more effective than vitamin C as a reducing agent for enhancing the utilization of iron, and the amino acids cystine and cysteine
- it helps prevent the harmful effects of high dose radiation, chemotherapy, x-rays, etc.
- it is an important amino acid transporter
- it accelerates respiration in the brain
- it helps protect against cigarette smoke and the poisoning effect of alcohol.

Although originally given by injection, a team of research scientists in Japan have concluded that glutathione, given orally, is very efficiently absorbed into the bloodstream.

Free radicals are thought to be the source of another aging indication, that is "cross linking." That process leads to tightening and shrinking of the collagen in your body leading to leathery and wrinkled skin.

Also, it leads to arteries that lose their ability to freely expand and contract and to joints that stiffen.

Glutathione's synergism with the antioxidant nutrients Vitamin E and selenium has attracted much experimental interest in aging research and many projects are now underway to discover that cause and effect relationship.

As mentioned previously, cell membranes contain fats and they are very susceptible to free radical damage. They are turned rancid. Think of the fat on meat that has turned rancid after too many days in the fridge or too many hours outside the fridge. Think of the way it looks and smells.

That's what I mean by rancid, *and it can happen inside the body!* Not a very happy thought but it's one of the problems of aging.

The main symptoms of excess free radicals include heart disease, liver disease, skin diseases, age spots, wrinkling, and so on.

Glutathione peroxidase prevents destruction of cell membranes by removing several classes of those peroxides.

When you look for free radical fighters in the health food store or your drug store, look for a combination of SOD and catalase and, if there's some glutathione peroxidase thrown in, so much the better. Follow label directions and make sure that the tablets are enteric coated.

More About Cells Getting Older and the Antioxidant Glutathione

Cells become aged, run out of energy and die.

That's all of us in a nutshell.

But we'd like to delay that event and enjoy our longer life.

When there is an absence of any particular essential amino acid, vitamin, mineral, or any essential element, the cell functions will be slowed, causing the cell to age more rapidly.

Everything that concerns the organism (you) concerns your cells. That includes stress, pollution, diet, drug therapies. . . even an argument with your spouse will knock off a few cells.

Some substances help the cell regenerate, that's why we've been talking about antioxidants. Glutathione was discovered back in 1921 by a researcher named Hopkins. He found it to be a unique sulfur-containing amino acid made from L-cysteine, L-glutamic acid, and glycine. Physicians gave it only by injection when it was first discovered, but now it can be used orally.

Research conducted at Harvard Medical School confirmed its antioxidant power and also that it protects your lungs against dust and harmful bacteria.

When glutathione teams up with the selenium-containing enzyme glutathione peroxidase, it directly deactivates free radicals. It also aids in detoxification by forming conjugates with heavy metals like lead, cadmium and mercury. This helps detoxify blood-pressure-elevating heavy metals and many other harmful substances.

Of special interest is the liver protection provided by glutathione against the effects of alcohol.

An article published in Science in 1981 indicated that glutathione destroyed aflatoxin-induced liver cancer in laboratory rats.

NOTE: When cells age they lose some of their glutathione content, as much as 30 percent, so supplement.

Glutathione's synergism with the antioxidant nutrients Vitamin E and selenium has attracted much experimental interest in aging research and many projects are now underway to discover the cause and effect relationship.

The Methione Reductase Enzyme

This is new. It was discovered by biochemists specializing in plant genetics. It is an enzyme that neutralizes the hydroxyl radical, the main radical generated by exposure to radiation.

Radiation is not the only source of the hydroxyl radical. Strenuous exercise is another! Loads of radicals are formed when we exercise in a closed room or in a polluted atmosphere. Think of all the joggers running along in traffic. They may be doing more harm than good to their body.

After exercise they have to clean out the extra metabolic waste material they've accumulated. The hydroxyl radicals are created when we burn fat for fuel. We want to burn fat during exercise and during dieting but we also want to take out the garbage.

Also, when we burn fat, we liberate the toxins and chemicals the body has stored away in those lumps of fat.

Catch 22. It's good to get rid of fat. We need it for energy to exercise so we can slim down and feel better and younger. But, when we burn the fat we let loose destructive material in the body that can do damage to the cells.

What's The Answer?

Exercise and take the supplements that can protect you against the danger, letting the toxins pass through your body like water. You may get some extra benefits as well. Athletes taking methione reductase report greater endurance, stamina, flexibility and a better ability to recover from hard workouts.

It may be a little hard to find but methione reductase is available from your health food store. Ask for it and if it's not on the shelf they can get it.

Follow label directions.

Pycnogenol — Most Powerful Antioxidant

In the winter of 1535, Jacques Cartier became the first European to visit what is now known as Canada. But tragedy was waiting for him and his crew. The iceflows in the waters off Quebec trapped his ship and his 110 companions, his supplies (limited to salt pork and biscuits), and they all fell victim to scurvy. Their teeth loosened and fell out, their gums bled, their bones became fragile and they hemorrhaged from their mucous membranes.

Twenty five died before a rescue party in the form of a group of Quebec Indians arrived with a gift of tea.

Not the tea we're accustomed to, but tea made from the bark of the Anneda pine tree.

Today, certain compounds in that tea — proanthocyanidins — are known to act as powerful antioxidants which scavenge and neutralize disease-causing free radical compounds.

Scurvy is caused by a deficiency in ascorbic acid (vitamin C). Bark from the Anneda pine tree contains ascorbic acid and, in addition, significant amounts of proanthocyanidins which are a form of bioflavonoid. The combination of vitamin C and the power of the bioflavonoids saved the lives of the French captain and the reaminder of his crew.

In the 1960's, Jack Masquelier, Ph.D., at the University of Bordeaux, France discovered that copious amounts of the same bioflavonoids were to be found in the bark of the maritime pine tree (Pinus maritima). He isolated the bioflavonoid, called it pycnogenol, and patented his findings. Laboratory evaluations and human testing have confirmed that pycnogenol is one of nature's most powerful antioxidants.

In the book, *The New Superantioxidant,* Keats Publishing, 1992, Richard Passwater, Ph.D. wrote that researchers at Nagasaki University School of Medicine found it was "fifty times more powerful than vitamin E in a test that measures the ability of compounds to scavenge free radicals."

"Health nuts" are well aware that vitamin E, along with vitamins A and C, represent some of the best antioxidants you can find in food and in supplements. For a reputable scientist like Dr.

Passwater to praise the action of pycnogenol in that manner is strong praise indeed for its action.

Most of the research has been done in Europe and the Orient where it has been determined that pycnogenol helps to retard the aging process.

How?

It stimulates blood circulation, improves vision, increases flexibility and reduces bruising. It may reduce the risk of cancer, heart disease and stroke, inflammation in arthritis, and help a number of other conditions.

Such A Powerful Substance Must Cause Serious Side Effects In Those Who Use It.

Not according to testing done at the Pasteur Institute in Lyon, France.

Their research has shown it to be nontoxic, noncarcinogenic and nonmutagenic. In plain language, it is safe!

Dr. Passwater states that people should begin taking between 100 and 150 mg daily, in divided doses, for several weeks and then switch to a maintenance dose of 50 mg daily.

Pycnogenol is not cheap but neither is good health.

Why Not Just Drink The Tea Made From The Bark That Saved Cartier And His Crew?

Probably a good idea but, so far, I haven't been able to find such a tea on the market.

The bioflavonoids in pycnogenol are also present in small amounts in beans, grapes, cranberries and some other forms of fruits and vegetables, but nowhere nearly as concentrated as that found in the pine.

So, once again, native medicine has proven itself. And there's so much more we have to learn about herbs.

Other Antioxidants

Nature works with combinations.

Briefly, here are some of the other nutrients you should be taking to combat age. We'll go into them more later in this book.

Vitamin E promotes the healthful use of oxygen while limiting the harmful "rusting" of cells caused by free radicals. Dr. Jeffry Bland has said that the lifespan of red blood cells could be extended several times past the fifty expected divisions if sufficient vitamin E were to be made available to the body.

Vitamin C stimulates the immune system which manufactures white blood cells, adrenal hormones, antibodies and interferon. The immune system deteriorates as we age, leading to infections and the degenerative diseases associated with old age.

Vitamin A protects epithelial tissue. Many of the human cancers that are found are epithelial cell malignancies. Vitamin A is especially efficient for scavenging the free radicals caused by cigarette smoke, chemicals and air pollution.

Selenium enhances the function of vitamin E and is part of the enzyme system which fights free radicals.

B-complex vitamins are stimulants to the immune system. According to the *American Journal of Clinical Nutrition* 46:659-664 (October 1987). Mary C. Talbott, et al. Oregon State University, Corvallis, Oregon, the authors suggest that improved vitamin B^6 nutriture in elderly persons may improve in vivo cell-mediated and humoral immunity, especially in those with poor vitamin B^6 status.

Gerontologists report that most people could both extend their lifespan and stay younger-looking much longer. The key to longer life may be an optimal intake of antioxidant and antiaging nutrients coupled to a moderate lifestyle and routine exercise.

What About Antioxidants And Cancer?

Cancer is certainly a frightening word because it is the second leading cause of death in the United States. At this time, 910,000 new cancers are diagnosed every year and it has been estimated that one of every four Americans will develop some form of cancer.

Cancer cells can be present in the body and not develop into life-threatening situations. They are born and then destroyed by the body's defense system.

Cancer is the common name for a large group of diseases that are characterized by the uncontrolled growth and spread of abnormal cells. Normally, the cells that make up the body reproduce themselves in an orderly way so worn-out tissues are replaced and injuries are repaired. Quite often cells change to a pre-cancerous state, but the body's immune system detects this change and destroys the abnormal cells. It is only when cells undergo abnormal change without detection by the immune system and begin a process of uncontrollable growth and spread that they may grow into masses of tissue (tumors). These can be either benign or malignant. Cancer invades and destroys normal tissue and, if left untreated, may result in death.

Cancer is believed to be the result of external factors combined with a hereditary disposition. A number of cancer-promoters have been identified in the diet and the environment. The estimate is that 75-80 percent of all human cancers are caused by the environment and about 30 to 40 percent by diet.

Free radical damage is thought to be involved in the initiation and promotion of many cancers. They are produced in the body, as said before. They come from smog, radiation, cigarette smoke and other environmental factors and, unless they are neutralized, they can cause considerable damage.

Not only do they interfere with a longer, more productive life, but they seem to increase in activity the longer we live.

Increased incidence of cancer may be due, at least in part, to the increasing level of free radical activities with longer age, plus the diminishing ability of the immune system to eliminate altered cells.

The use of antioxidants by older people can preserve their active lifestyle.

Cooperative Defense Systems

We've talked about the body's ability to defend itself. It's too bad it's not familiar with all of the poisons in the air, food and water. So many new poisons are made every year that the body has a hard time even recognizing what's a poison and what's a food.

Cooperative defense systems which attempt to protect the body against the cancer-damage of free radicals include certain enzymes (SOD, catalase, glutathione) and the antioxidant vitamins E, A, and C, the minerals selenium and zinc, and the amino acids methionine and cysteine.

The National Cancer Institute has funded 28 studies to investigate the association between antioxidants and cancer prevention and risk. Results of cell and animal research and limited epidemiological human studies suggest that the antioxidants alter cancer incidence by acting as anticarcinogens.

High intakes of vitamin E enhance the body's immune system and also protect vitamin A. Vitamins E and C keep smoked, pickled and cured foods from becoming cancer-causing in your stomach. Vitamin A stimulates the immune response and controls the growth, alteration and functions of body tissues. Selenium, in addition to its inclusion in the enzyme glutathione peroxidase, enhances immune response with potentially increased resistance to cancer initiation and growth.

Although it is gratifying to see that the National Cancer Institute is investigating the use of nutrients as cancer-fighters, it's strange that it does its investigating in body sections. Various medical institutions have been assigned separate body parts and different nutrients to investigate.

Here are some of the body areas, the institute researching them and the nutrients being tested.

Body area	Nutrients	Institution
Colon	Vitamin C and E	Dartmouth
"	Beta-carotene, C, E	"
"	C, E, Wheat bran	Memorial
"	13-cic retinoic acid	U. of W. Virginia
"	Beta-carotene	U. of Illinois
Digestive Tract	C, E	MIT
Cervix	Trans-retinoic acid	U. of Arizona
Esophagus	Beta-carotene	NCI, Maryland
"	Multiple vitamins and minerals	NCI, Maryland

It's not necessary to continue what and where, but you can see that the body has been divided into its parts. Lung, skin, breast, etc. have been assigned to other research institutions.

Meantime, while the public has not been advised of the role of a number of these nutrients as an aid to disease prevention and longer life, there have been articles written in the general press about beta-carotene and other nutrients. The main thrust of the articles and medical opinion is that nutrients can be obtained from the diet in sufficient amounts.

If that were so, then we wouldn't have the number of cancer deaths we have now!

Other than programs to decrease cigarette smoking, there are few areas of research that appear as promising to substantially reducing cancer incidence as nutritional supplementation.

Of course you have to eat better foods, and you have to exercise along with taking supplements.

The following recommendations of some antioxidants should be discussed with your nutritionally-oriented doctor:

Antioxidant	RDA	Recommendations	Possible Toxicity Level
Vitamin E	10-20 I.U.	200-800 I.U.	Negligible at less than 1200 I.U.
Vitamin A	5000 I.U.	12,500 I.U.	Limited (chronic intakes above 25,000 I.U.)
Vitamin C	60 mg	1,000 mg	Negligible at 1–2 grams
Selenium	none	50 - 200 mcg	Potential toxicity at over 200 mcg

Based on the increasing age-adjusted mortality rate associated with cancer, a shift from treatment to prevention seems necessary until the investigations into the benefits of antioxidants catch up to the reality that they can keep people living longer!

References

1. Passwater, R.A. *Supernutrition: Megavitamin Revolution.* 176-7 Dial Press, N.Y. (1975).
2. Tappel, A.L. *Geriatrics* 23(10) 102(1968).
3. Devlin, T.M. *Textbook of Biochemistry,* 1035, Wiley N.Y. (1982).
4. Hsu, J.M. *J. Nutr.* 111:26-33 (1981).
5. Sunderman, F.W. *Fed. Proc.* 37:40-46 (1978).
6. Maines, M.D. *Proc. Natl. Acad. Sci.,* 74:1875-8 (1977).
7. Lemen, R.A. *Ann. N.Y. Acad. Sci.,* 271-273-9 (1976).
8. Sprince, H., et al. *Fed. Proc.* 33(3) 102 (1974).
9. Sies, H. and Wendel, A. *Functions of Glutathione,* 189, Springer-Verlag, N.Y. (1978).
10. Green, G.M. *Science* 162-810-11 (1968).
11. Novi, A.M. *Science* 212-541-2 (1981).
12. Hazelton, G.A. *Biochem. J.,* 188-25-30 (1980).
13. Lacour, B., et al. *Lancet,* ii, 763, 1980.
14. Fraenkel, G. and Friedman, S. *Vitamins and Hormones* 16:73, 1957.
15. Carter, H.E., et al. *Arch. Biochem. Biophys.* 36:405, 1952.
16. Askew, E.W., et al. *Nutr. Metab.* 24:32, 1980.
17. Novak, M., et al. *Bio. Neonate* 25:85, 1975.
18. Suzuki, M., et al. *J. Nutr. Sci. Vitaminol.* 22:169, 1976.
19. Holloszy, J. *Exercise Sports Sci. Rev.* 1:45, 1973.
20. Tsai, A.C., et al. *J. Nutr.* 104:782, 1974.
21. Mole, P.A., et al. *J. Clin. Invest.* 50:2323, 1971.
22. Hahn, P., et al. *Can. J. Physiol. Pharmacol* 49:853, 1971.
23. Whitaker, J., et al. *Am. J. Med.* 63:805, 1977.
24. Angelini, C., et al. *Neurology* 26:633, 1976.
25. Hosein, E. *Biochem. Pharm.* 24:1859, 1975.
26. Maebashi, M., et al. *Lancet,* ii, 805, 1978.

Dimethylaminoethanol

Let's call it DMAE for short.

It's a natural product found in large quantities in what grandma called "brain food." Fish such as sardines and anchovies are loaded with it.

It stimulates the production of choline and acetylcholine in the brain. They're the neurotransmitters involved in learning, memory, movement, and sensory functions.

DMAE is one of the memory enhancing substances that appear to be of great potential in the area of life enhancement and extension. The body and the brain are one and both must be healthy for life's enjoyment.

DMAE is the immediate precursor to choline in the building and repair of cellular membrane, especially in the brain and the nervous system. DMAE makes choline and it is choline inside the cells that is then converted into phosphatidyl choline and then into cell membrane. What is most important is that this conversion takes place within the area where it is most needed and does not have to wait for dietary choline to be transported to the area.

The Good Part

DMAE treated mice lived 30 percent longer than untreated mice.

The Bad Part

DMAE is tough to find. It is part of some vitamin formulas but you'll have to search for it because the FDA doesn't believe it has redeeming qualities.

Glandulars (Cell Therapy)

Way back when, physicians believed that "like heals like."

If the heart is in trouble, feed the patient heart. If the lungs are in trouble, feed the patient lung.

The concept then was that the healthy cell would migrate to the unhealthy cell and stimulate its own power to heal and revitalize itself.

Doctors who practice cell therapy believe it resembles an organ transplant without the operation, and actually is able to make old cells "act younger."

Modern cell healing or therapy was re-discovered in 1931 by a Swiss physician Paul Niehans. His concept was to inject fresh glandulars into patients, with the effect lasting longer than any synthetic hormone, implant or surgical graft.

Dr. Niehans has said that his aim is to give more years to life and more life to years. He says his aim was to make all the organs struck by old age capable once more of functioning properly and, at the same time, to bring fresh strength to the whole body by revitalizing the sex glands.

Cell therapy is designed to solve the following:

- loss of vitality
- physical and mental exhaustion
- premature aging
- signs of deterioration of organs
- lack of drive
- declining mental efficiency
- weakness of the immune system

What Actually Is Cell Therapy?

It is an implantation by injection of animal origin, fetal or juvenile suspension of cells or tissues in physiological solution. It's like transplanting an organ but, instead of the entire organ being surgically transplanted, the cells of the organ are used.

The transplanted cell then somehow brings about a revitalization of the corresponding organ.

All other civilized countries of the world accept this concept, but the United States and Canada do not.

Cell therapy as done by Niehans is not available in the U.S. It is available in Europe and in Mexico.

The late actor Steve McQueen received alternative treatment for terminal mesothelioma, a rare form of cancer, and live cell injections were part of his treatment at the American Biologics — Mexico Hospital. He entered the hospital in the summer of 1980 after his doctors in America had given him no more than two weeks to live. He survived, and four months later was improving.

Then, against the advice of his doctors in Mexico, he went to another clinic for removal of tumors by surgery. . . and died of an embolism following the operation.

Live cell therapy has been sought out by other famous people, including Charles Chaplin, President Eisenhower, Bernard Baruch, Joseph Kennedy, Pablo Picasso, Noel Coward and many others.

Although not allowed in this country, there has been research done on the theory. Professor Paul Weiss of the Rockefeller Institute conducted experiments which showed that single cells are equipped with a "self-organizing" capacity so that certain information contained within specific cells reacts in such a way that masses of cells become identifiable as tissues. For example, heart cells link to one another to form rhythmically contracting tissue. The reasoning behind cell therapy is the normalizing of hormones — their harmonizing effect — and the build-up of damaged tissues leading to their rejuvenation.

But If We Cannot Get This Therapy, Why The Information?

Historically, glandulars are not completely unfamiliar to us. Injecting glands into the system may be, but glands as food are not. When eating meat, most primitive people and animals eat the entire food source, including the internal organs, glands and muscle tissue. This makes a lot of sense since glands and organs vary in their nutritional content. Zinc, for example, is extremely high in the prostate gland, but low in any other organ.

There was a time when Americans regularly ate heart, stomach, pancreas, thymus glands and even brains. Today, we have a tendency to eat only the muscle meats of cattle, hogs and chickens. French cuisine still makes use of other parts, but Americans have lost the know-how to cook them.

It can be made easy with a little common sense, if not haute cuisine. To ground beef, a typical staple on American tables, add one quarter by weight of organ meat. The taste remains the same, but the nutrition is raised.

Or, if the concept of eating glands is still not appealing, consider the use of glandular tablets or capsules.

Several firms manufacture tablets that contain concentrates of raw glands. They are available at your health food store and even at drug counters in some areas.

It is possible that raw glandular extracts will improve the efficiency of our own similar glands.

Which Glands Are Available?

- The Pituitary
- The Adrenals
- The Thymus
- The Pancreas
- The Spleen
- The Heart
- The Testes
- The Ovary
- The Parotids

Do not limit your search for rejuvenation to glandulars alone. Combine it with vitamin therapies, diet, exercise and other nutrients.

5

VITAMINS AGAINST AGING

I have no quarrel with the FDA.

They say that the RDA (Recommended Daily Allowance) of vitamins is sufficient to prevent symptoms of deficiency to appear in normal Americans who eat a balanced diet.

I buy that. The RDA will be enough to prevent symptoms if you are normal, if you eat a balanced diet, and if the vitamins are present in that normal diet.

But, who is normal?

What's a balanced diet?

Who labels food with the vitamin content and who tested the food?

And, most important of all, who wants to live just on the edge of showing deficiency symptoms?

If the body needs just so much of vitamins to keep it from being sick, shouldn't it benefit from a higher level of those vitamins?

This chapter is about using more than just the RDA of vitamins to improve the chances of living longer and better. We won't go into all the uses of vitamins, only those which impact upon life extension.

Although we know many of the biochemical roles for vitamins, we don't know all there is to know about them. Investigations will continue but if we wait for all the news to be in, some of us will not be around to benefit. The FDA has established the RDA for all the essential vitamins. Lately, there has been a tendency to use megadoses of them, up to hundreds of times the RDA. Although most nutritionists feel that up to ten times the RDA is a safe level, more daily dosage than that is in the realm of the unknown.

Vitamins should be taken in prudent amounts, and your body can advise you about prudence, because overdosing will result in unpleasant symptoms. If you experience problems, cut the dose down to a more comfortable level.

Vitamin A and Beta-Carotene

Cancer shortens life. Vitamin A and/or beta-carotene can help to prevent certain types of cancer. Scientific papers relating to these nutrients and their life-sparing attributes have appeared in both the scientific press and the lay press.

Vitamin A and beta-carotene are essential for human health and now they have been clearly established as life-savers.

What's The Difference Between Them?

Vitamin A is an oil soluble vitamin obtained from animals (mostly in the form of fish liver oil). It is ready to be absorbed since the animal has converted the source of the vitamin into vitamin A. Because it is oil soluble, it can be stored in the body. Many traditionalists point to vitamin A when they wish to scare people with stories of the dangers inherent in large amounts of vitamins for supplementation. Those scaremongers point to the one proven story of an explorer who died after eating the liver of a polar bear. What they fail to state is that polar bear liver contains on average about 1,500,000 units of vitamin A. Most people take between 5,000 and 20,000 units of the vitamin. So, if you're in the Arctic and stop in at a native restaurant, don't order polar bear liver, and, if you do, eat only a miniscule portion.

Bete-carotene is found in plants and not in animals. It is two molecules of vitamin A linked together. As long as the links remain whole, beta-carotene does not have vitamin A activity. When the body needs vitamin A, it releases an enzyme which cuts the link and separates the two molecules. Then there is vitamin A activity.

Because of the linkage, there is no chance of a vitamin A overdose, so those people who have been afraid to take vitamin A, because they were impressed by the story about its toxicity and didn't know about the polar bear, can take beta-carotene without worry.

In a nutshell, vitamin A is ready to use and is stored in the body, but may be a problem if a super-large dose is used. Beta-carotene must be unlocked by the body and cannot be harmful.

NOTE: MANY DIABETICS CANNOT UNLOCK THE LINKAGE OF BETA-CAROTENE AND HAVE TO USE THE REGULAR VITAMIN A.

Do They Act In The Same Way?

Yes, but the beta-carotene has additional protective power.

All vitamin A substances appear to be protective against some types of cancers. Vitamin A, from fish or from plants, is necessary for night vision, regulation of cell development, reproduction and the health of all epithelial tissue and mucous membrane. When it is deficient, alterations in the skin and the mucous membrane begin to resemble precancerous tissue.

Carotenoids have been shown to have anti-cancer effects in mice and rats. What helps them usually helps us.

(*Science,* 221:1256, 1983)

Concerning scientific studies on toxicity, patients were given 300 milligrams or 500,000 International Units of beta-carotene for prolonged periods and showed no toxic effects.

(*Archives of Dermatology,* 113:1229, 1977)

One of the ways beta-carotene works is to quench a destructive form of oxygen called singlet oxygen. This form of oxygen is toxic to the individual cells. Beta-carotene acts at the tissue level to quench the fire of singlet oxygen.

(*Nature,* 290:201, 1981)

One thing that must be made clear is that vitamin A or beta-carotene can never be substituted for good health habits. You can't continue to smoke cigarettes and take supplements to ward off the ill effects. That's only fooling yourself. If you *stop* smoking and take supplements you're on your way to longer life.

The smoking habits and the eating habits of more than 8,000 Norwegian men were studied over a period of five years. The smokers with the lowest intake of beta-carotene showed the highest incidence of cancer, particularly lung cancer.

(*International Journal of Cancer*, 15:561, 1975)

A similar study of about 2,000 men in Chicago over a nineteen-year period made a finding which coincided with the Norwegian study. Smokers with the lowest intake of beta-carotene were more likely to develop lung cancer.

(*Lancet*, 2:1185, 1981)

But it is not only in the lungs and with smokers that beta-carotene has shown its ability to ward off problems. The reader can obtain the following publications and read the reports for themselves:

- *Journal of the National Cancer Institute*, 62:1435, 1979 — the bladder.
- *American Journal of Epidemiology*, 113:675, 1981 — the larynx.
- *Nutrition and Cancer*, 2:143, 1981 — the esophagus.

And there's more about the effects of beta-carotene on the stomach, the prostate, the colon and rectum, etc.

If you can get a copy of, "Selected Abstracts on Vitamin A and Cancer Biology," National Cancer Institute, Bethesda, 1979, you can read for yourself all of the papers demonstrating how vitamin A and beta-carotene can suppress the malignant behavior of body cells.

It's Impressive. What Else Do Vitamin A And Beta-Carotene Do?

Cancer is not the only factor that shortens life. Infections can do the same thing. We've all known people who have succumbed to bacterial or viral infections. When there is a deficiency of vitamin A, the mucous membrane (it covers the inside of the nose, mouth, lungs, vaginal tract, etc.) cannot function the way it should. It dries and cracks and permits the entrance of germs and viruses of all types.

(*Nutrition and the M.D.*, 8:1, 1982)

Vitamin A and beta-carotene also help in healing wounds, boosting immunity, and fighting skin diseases.

How Can We Get Enough Of Each?

You can eat calf's liver. A half-pound serving will give you about 75,000 I.U., while a large sweet potato will contain almost 10,000 I.U. of beta-carotene. Also, eat carrots, broccoli, spinach, collards, kale, cantaloupe, mustard greens, papayas, apricots, tomatoes, watermelons.

Take supplements of beta-carotene, 15,000 to 25,000 I.U., or take vitamin A in doses of from 5,000 to 15,000 I.U.

Some people will want to take more supplements because their eating habits don't provide enough natural vitamin A and/or beta-carotene. Or, they may work with hazardous chemicals or in a smoke-filled atmosphere. If you have to go above the recommended dose, try to find a nutritionally-oriented M.D. and work it out with him or her.

Most drug stores and health food stores have both the regular A and the beta-carotene. Many vitamin/mineral formulas will contain both, so check the label carefully for their presence and to see what amounts are contained.

Beta-carotene should be used as a supplement for other reasons other than its action against free radicals. Besides its antioxidant activity, it appears that it may also be able to enhance the body's immune function.

It has been shown to increase macrophage production of tumor necrosis factor (TNF) and the T-Helper cell stimulator, interleukin 1. This shows activity in a direct way against destructive body cells which shorten your lifespan.

Many people are adversely affected by prolonged exposure to the sun. Non-melanoma cancer of the skin is now the most common form of cancer among the white population of the United States. A pathological sensitivity to light, called photosensitization, can be triggered in susceptible persons by drugs, cosmetics, or many environmental chemicals. Beta-carotene may be able to offer protection to those individuals and act as a buffer against skin damage from the sun.

The diets of a group of healthy women, and also those with abnormal PAP smears suggesting the risk of cancer, were examined by Dr. Wylie-Rosett and her colleagues at the Albert Einstein College of Medicine. The study showed that women with higher beta-carotene intake from their diets had a threefold lower risk of developing the cancer, cervical dysplasia.

(*Nutrition and Cancer*, Vol. 6, No. 1, 1984)

According to Dr. Eli Seifter, professor of biology, chemistry, and surgery at the same college, referring to his tests with animals, beta-carotene — in a sense — is a "morning after pill." Even after exposure to cancer-producing doses of some toxic chemicals, beta-carotene still has its effect. He likes a daily intake of 5 to 10 milligrams, the equivalent of 8,375 to 16,750 I.U. of vitamin A, normally, and perhaps twice that amount for high risk people like smokers.

Beta-Carotene Shrinks Tumors

According to an article in *Prescription Drug News*, Vol. 2, No. 7, 1987, which referred to a study published in *Carcinogenesis* documenting research done at Harvard University:

Cancerous tumors in the mouth can be reduced or prevented by carotene.

According to the study, cancerous tumors in the mouths of hamsters disappeared within two weeks after being injected in the mouth with beta-carotene or having a beta-carotene solution applied directly to the tumor.

While other research has shown that people who eat fruits and vegetables high in beta-carotene seem to have a lower incidence of cancer, this is the first study that examined the effects of injecting or applying carotene to existing cancerous tumors!

Cholesterol-Lowering Vitamin B^3 Lowers the Mortality Rate

The increased intake of niacin (vitamin B^3) has been shown to lower the death rate of men who have previously suffered heart attacks.

What a great thing to know. An inexpensive vitamin may be able to extend life! And do it better than diet alone, or any one of five commonly prescribed drugs.

According to a report in *The Medical Tribune,* February 19, 1986, niacin got a negative reputation with the medical profession because of the bad side effects associated with its use. The original studies in the large-scale Coronary Drug Project used 7 to 8 grams a day. This ten-year study involved 8,000 men who had previously had a heart attack. Although the study showed the superiority of niacin over other treatments, the side effects experienced by the men given niacin made its use unacceptable.

So Why Raise Our Hopes?

A new study indicates that the niacin advantage can be obtained in much lower doses. Dr. James D. Alderman, senior fellow in cardiology at Boston's Beth Israel Hospital gave 1 to 2 grams of niacin daily to 72 men and women with documented coronary heart disease, 34 of whom had had heart attacks. They started out with 100 milligrams a day, with most reaching the 2 gram dosage (2,000 milligrams) as they were able to tolerate it.

The patients reported dramatic reduction in the ratio of total cholesterol to HDL (high density lipoprotein or "good cholesterol." The Framington Heart Study has demonstrated that the reduction in the ratio of total cholesterol to HDL ratio *reduces* the risk of heart attack; it has a far greater impact than the reduction of total cholesterol alone.

Dr. Alderman said that niacin may offer more lipid-lowering benefits than traditional medication or diet alone at a much lower cost.

What Are The Side Effects Of Using Niacin?

Niacin can cause what is called the "flush reaction." Because it is able to dilate blood vessels, the face, head, arms and hands, and even the chest can become very red. The area feels warm to hot and sometimes causes a prickly or tingling feeling. It's not dangerous but it can be scary.

One of the ways this flush reaction can be minimized or negated altogether is to take niacin in a time-release form. Usually it is available in a 500 milligram tablet that will release the niacin slowly, only as fast as it can be absorbed by the body.

Its benefits will be forthcoming after about two months of vitamin therapy. Check with your doctor about using niacin.

Niacin may be able to reverse atherosclerosis (*New England Journal of Medicine*, 304:251, 1981).

Where Can We Get It?

All health food stores and all drug stores, but since all time-release tablets may not be truly time-release, ask if there have been blood studies done to check the rate of release of the vitamin.

For normal use, niacin or niacinamide is usually a part of the B-Complex group found in a multiple vitamin/mineral formula. 15 to 50 milligrams daily is the usual dose. Or check the label for directions.

Another Plus for Niacin (Vitamin B^3)

Niacin appears to have other anti-aging powers besides its ability to help reduce serum cholesterol levels.

It hold strong promise in cancer prevention and may also have value in treatment of the disease.

Based on findings presented by nearly 200 of the world's leading scientists in the area of niacin nutrition and cancer during an international symposium at the Texas College of Osteopathic Medicine.

Research indicates that niacin, through its activities in cellular repair, may serve a role in cancer prevention. Dr. Myron K. Jacobson and Dr. Elaine Jacobson, Ph.D's. demonstrated that cells deficient in niacin develop cancer at a rate that is ten times greater than cells with sufficient amounts of the vitamin.

The difficulty is in determining the optimal amount of niacin people should take. The current RDA is 20 milligrams and that's the least people should take. Eggs, nuts, peanut butter, whole grains, wheat germ and brewer's yeast will supply some of the vitamin.

The general conclusion drawn from the four-day meeting (International Symposium on ADP-Ribosylation) was that niacin is essential in repair to cellular DNA. The vitamin is converted to NAD in the body and NAD regulates many more mechanisms than previously thought.

NOTE: As more research into nutrition is made public, the notion that prevention of disease is the key to longer life will become more and more "the way to go!"

The Anti-Stress Factor Vitamin from the B-Complex Group — B^6

(*American Journal of Clinical Nutrition* 46: 659-664, October 1987)

Stress can shorten your life!

Vitamin B^6 is a member of the B-Complex group of vitamins. This group is frequently called the "nerve complex" group because, for those of you who suffer from stress and the accompanying physical symptoms, this group may be the most important supplement you can add to your daily diet routine.

While most Americans are aware of the importance of a well-balanced diet complete with proper amounts of vitamins, minerals and accessory nutrients essential to good health, they are not as aware of the particular vitamins which can contribute to a longer life. Vitamin B^6 is one of them.

The elderly tend to have lower vitamin B^6 status than younger people. There was a study done to see if increasing the B^6 intake would increase the immune status of older people. The subjects were from 65 to 81 years of age and they were given 50 milligrams of B^6 a day.

The result was a stimulated immune response and therefore better protection to the body.

Vitamins are necessary in the diet to promote normal growth and maintain normal life functions. They are natural components of enzyme systems required for cellular activity — organic compounds which are necessary for the normal growth and maintenance of body tissues. When they are not present in adequate amounts, a deficiency disease will develop.

A number of reasons exist for a deficiency, including:

- Inadequate dietary or supplementary intake
- Poor absorption and utilization of the vitamin

- Increased loss due to excretion or to interference from drugs
- Increased need

Vitamins are either water soluble and unable to be stored in the body, or fat soluble and able to be stored. The B-Complex is water soluble and is needed on a daily basis.

When the B-vitamins are in short supply, the symptoms usually include personality changes, apprehensiveness, moodiness and worry. But these are only symptoms for others to notice, since the subject usually ignores them.

Among other benefits, the B-Complex has been attributed with:

- Providing energy and well-being
- Acting as a natural tranquilizer
- Helping to relieve fatigue and insomnia
- Relieving irritability
- Providing an "extra lift" so you can get through the day without killing yourself or someone else

Vitamin B^6 (pyridoxine) was isolated and named in 1939. Its primary job in the body is to produce certain hormones, hemoglobins, and other compounds which are necessary for the normal functioning of the brain and the nerves. It is necessary to the utilization of protein and the growth and maintenance of body functions. It also:

- Assimilates proteins and fats
- Aids in the conversion of the amino acid tryptophan into niacin
- Helps prevent various nerve and skin disorders
- Alleviates nausea
- Promotes the proper synthesis of *anti-aging* nucleic acids
- Reduces night muscle spasms, leg cramps, hand numbness and certain forms of neuritis in the extremities
- Works as a natural diuretic

Researchers at the University of Wisconsin in Madison suggest that vitamin B^6 may be useful in treating cancer. Dr. David Rose, the endocrinologist in charge of the study, suggests that B^6 might be beneficial to women with breast cancer who have been found to be deficient.

Other physicians theorize that arteriosclerosis may be a result of the metabolism of an amino acid into homocysteine. The use of B^6 in a daily intake of 10 to 25 milligrams daily (5 to 10 times the RDA) will keep your arteries flexible and clear. (You can consult your physician for the dose best for you.)

Although vitamin B^6 is found in liver, whole grain cereals, potatoes, red meat, vegetables and corn, as well as Brewer's yeast, wheat bran, cabbage, milk, beets and cantaloupe, these points must be taken into consideration.

- It is easily destroyed by heat (cooking, for example).
- If you eat a lot of protein you need much more B^6 in your diet.
- B^6 is water soluble and is lost within 8 hours after taking. This means you need a time-release supplement or you should take your supplement 2 to 3 times a day in divided doses.
- An excess of choline can mean you need more B^6 as a balance.
- B^6 works best with B^1, B^2, pantothenic acid, vitamin C, niacin or niacinamide, biotin, folic acid, and magnesium.
- If you're pregnant, check with your doctor before taking sustained doses of B^6.
- B^6 should not be taken by anyone under L-dopa treatment for Parkinson's disease.
- B^6 is destroyed by overcooking, long storage, canning, food processing, alcohol, and estrogens.

B^6 and PMS

Although not life threatening, many women wish they were dead when they suffer the symptoms of premenstrual tension. This syndrome has been attributed to a number of causes, some of

them hormonal. A study using vitamin B^6 in a powerful dose of 500 milligrams a day in time-release form reported that 21 out of 25 women in the study reported significant relief.
(*Infertility*, 3:155, 1980)

B^6 and Diabetes

There is some evidence, not conclusive, that some forms of this life-shortening disease may be contributed to by a B^6 deficiency.
(*Lancet*, April 10, 1976, pp. 788-789)

Because adequate levels of B^6 are required for the proper metabolism of the amino acid tryptophan, and abnormalities of tryptophan metabolism may contribute to glucose intolerance, supplemental B^6 may help to reverse the condition.
(*Journal of Clinical Investigation*, 40:617. 1961)

Also, supplementation with the vitamin may reduce the need for insulin in some diabetics.
(*Journal of Medicine*, Bordeaux, 138:881, 1961)

B^6 Boosts Immunity

Both animals and human volunteers subjected to deliberate B^6 depletion went into profound depression of cell-mediated and humoral-mediated immune functions. *Vitamin B^6 appears to be the most important of all of the B-vitamins for the normal functioning of the immune system.*

Several disease states are characteristically associated with immune-function deficiencies, for example certain types of cancer and AIDS (acquired immune deficiency syndrome).
(*American Journal of Clinical Nutrition*, 35: Feb. Supplement 1982, pp. 418-421)

B^6 Against Cancer

B^6 can inhibit the growth of a number of different types of cancer cells in culture.
(Disorbo and colleagues, *Nutrition and Cancer*, 5:10, 1983)

Where Do I Get It And How Much?

It is available in all health food stores and drug stores. It is a part of all of the B-Complex tablets and formulas and is also available separately.

How much you should take is another story. The FDA's RDA is 2 milligrams a day. Most people should not take more than 50 milligrams a day unless advised by their doctor.

The best thing would be to eat vitamin B^6 loaded foods and supplement for good measure.

About Vitamin B^6 and Osteoporosis

According to Dr. Alan Gaby, M.D. in his book, *B^6 The Natural Healer*, Keats Publishing, New Caanan, Conn., 1987, more than 30 percent of American women develop bone loss after menopause. Millions each year fracture their spine or hip as a result.

Numerous factors have been suggested as possible contributors to this situation and a great deal of calcium has been sold as a result. Both dietary calcium and supplemental calcium — with or without a vitamin D — are being prescribed by doctors or taken on their own by millions of women and men.

Also implicated is excess sugar consumption, excess animal protein, caffeine, alcohol, as well as a lack of exercise. However, outside of Dr. Gaby's book, I have not heard of a deficiency of vitamin B^6 as a possible cause of osteoporosis.

Except that it makes a great deal of sense.

Animals raised on diets low in vitamin B^6 have thinner bones than those fed a normal diet!

Since the average American diet is low in vitamin B^6, it seems prudent to listen to Dr. Gaby and insure an adequate amount by taking a supplemental B-Complex formula.

How much? As told in other parts of this book, up to 50 mg/day.

Pantothenic Acid (Calcium Pantothenate)

This vitamin is also a part of the B-Complex group and plays a number of essential roles in the metabolic process. It helps in the production of energy and is vital to the production of hormones from the adrenal glands.

As early as 1950, it was noted that when rats were deficient in this vitamin there were defects in the development and growth of bone and cartilage.

These defects were corrected when supplemental pantothenic acid was introduced into the diet.

This correction has led to the idea that pantothenic acid might be of substantial help in the treatment of human bone and joint disorders.

(Nelson et al. *Proceedings of the Society for Experimental Biology and Medicine,* 73:31, 1950)

Thirteen years later, Barton-Wright and Elliot (*Lancet,* 2:862, 1963) found that people suffering from rheumatoid arthritis had much lower pantothenic acid content in their body. When supplements of 50 milligrams a day were given, many of the systems were relieved. Best results were achieved with patients who were vegetarians and were given the fanciful combination of pantothenic acid and royal jelly. Royal jelly, the substance which is fed to regular bees to make a queen, is naturally high in pantothenic acid.

I've Heard That Pantothenic Acid Is An Energy Booster.

Many athletes do use it for energy and to boost athletic capability. Pantothenic acid can increase resistance to stress as shown by an animal study done in the early fifties. Rats given pantothenic acid were able to survive twice as long as unsupplemented rats when forced to remain in ice cold water. (*Vitamins and Hormones,* 11:133, 1953)

What About "Aging?"

There is a marvelous book written in 1971 (*Nutrition Against Disease,* Pitman, New York, 1971) by Dr. R.J. Williams who discovered pantothenic acid. In it he described his research in which laboratory animals, supplemented with pantothenic acid, lived up to 20 percent longer than mice and other animals that did not take the vitamin in supplemental form.

Therefore, it is possible that doses of pantothenic acid in amounts that are up to ten times the RDA can retard and remove age pigments on your skin, re-energize old cells and extend life span.

The RDA for pantothenic acid is 10 milligrams a day for adults.

Wound Healing and Pantothenic Acid (B^5)

The rapid healing of wounds is an indication of the internal health and youthfulness of an individual. Scientists have been investigating the nutritional requirements for wound healing for years. They've found that certain nutrients, including vitamin C and the amino acid methionine play important roles in the formation of collagen, the intercellular protein that constitutes the main component of the fabric of regenerated tissue. They've also discovered that the amino acids arginine and ornithine are capable of accelerating the wound-healing process.

Now there is new evidence that pantothenic acid (vitamin B^5) also can speed up healing. Scientists used rabbits for their research and found that pantothenic acid supplementation induced a "remarkable increase" in wound-healing ability.

(Aprahamian, Marc et al., *American Journal of Clinical Nutrition,* 41:578-589, 1985)

Pantothenic acid also has a potent anti-stress effect and can lower cholesterol levels.

Vitamin C and Longevity – Among Other Things

Vitamin C is the one vitamin all America knows.

But all America connects vitamin C with colds and flu and knows little more about its ability to fight cancer, combat cardiovascular disease, speed wound healing, protect against various diseases, and so on.

The protective effects of vitamin C against various types of cancers have been noted in a wide variety of studies:

The relationship between high cancer rates and low vitamin C intake (*Cancer Research,* 35:3452, 1975) and (*American Journal of Clinical Nutrition,* 34:2478, 1981).

See also: *American Journal of Epidemiology,* 114:714, 1981.
Internal Medicine News, 16 (No. 10) 49, 1983.

Studies suggest that vitamin C, because it is a powerful antioxidant, can block the formation of various cancer-causing substances, such as nitrosamines, in the body.

Although nitrosamine formation is usually linked to smoke-cured meat and nitrate-cured meat (bacon, ham, etc.) it is also present in cigarette smoke, beer, some cosmetics and even impure *drinking water*.

ONE GRAM OF VITAMIN C TAKEN DAILY HAS BEEN SHOWN TO BLOCK THE FORMATION OF SOME OF THESE SUBSTANCES IN THE BODY.
(*Cancer Research*, 40:1062, 1980)

What About The Common Cold?

The immune system, particularly the disease-fighting white blood cells, are very needful of a sufficient supply of vitamin C to carry out their normal functions. Since the level of vitamin C in the body is reduced during colds, infection, surgery, pregnancy, and other STRESSFUL situations, it is logical to assume that supplementation of vitamin C — either from the diet or from supplemental tablets or capsules — will help the immune system.

Stress, of any kind, will cause the vitamin C in the body to be used up.

Do you find that you are apt to get a cold after a violent argument with your spouse or your boss?

If you do, it might be a good idea to take some vitamin C whenever the situation arises. Same thing if your kid wrecks your car driving out of the garage!

Does Vitamin C Ward Off Viruses As Well As Help With A Cold?

Although there is a lot of controversy about vitamin C and colds and its other protective effects, I and a lot of researchers take it regularly.

High doses of vitamin C (above one gram daily) can boost the production and activity of interferon. Interferon is a natural virus-fighting substance produced by the body. When a virus invades the body it is unable to reproduce by itself. It must go into a cell and instruct the DNA in the cell to make another virus. Interferon is manufactured by an adjoining cell. Interferon cannot harm the virus but can go around to neighboring cells and tell the cells to change the composition of their walls so the virus will not be able to enter. The more interferon in the body the quicker the message will be spread around. If the virus cannot force the cells to make new viruses and the number of viruses is kept to a minimum, it will be easier for the white blood cells to engulf and destroy them.

(*Infection and Immunity*, 10:409, 1974)

Vitamin C research continues to point up its ability to enhance the immune function. When young adults were give 2 to 3 grams of vitamin C, neutrophils (white blood cells) became more active against invading bacteria or viruses.

(*American Journal of Clinical Nutrition*, 35:423, 1982)

Vitamin C Is Even Good for Your Teeth!

What do teeth have to do with longevity?

You have to chew your food before it can be digested.

You have to digest it before you can get the nutrients into your system.

Supplements alone will not do the trick. You need nutrients from food as well.

Although many people do not have cavities the way they did in past years, gum disease is more prevalent than it has been.

Recently, researchers at the University of Texas have found that vitamin C can prevent gum disease in many cases.

(*American Health*, Sept./Oct. 1983, p.31)

Cardiovascular Research

Vitamin C works against blood clots.

(*Thrombosis Review*, 15:639, 1979)

(*Atherosclerosis*, 35:181, 1980)

It has also been found that many individuals suffering from atherosclerosis have low levels of vitamin C in their bodies.

(*Journal of Nutrition*, 99:261, 1969)

How Much Should I Take?

That's a tough question because the need for vitamin C will vary with the individual, his or her lifestyle, the environment, diet, cigarettes and alcohol, age, etc.

I take 1,000 to 1,500 milligrams a day.

The Better To See You My Dear

Diets that are high in folic acid and vitamin C are associated with a reduced risk for cataracts, the number one cause of dim eyesight in old age.

What's the good of taking care of your immune system, adding years to your life, and having problems with your eyesight?

Food frequency questionnaires and supplement data was obtained from 78 patients who suffered from cataracts in at least one eye. The diets were analyzed for concentrations of vitamins A, B^1, B^2, B^6, B^{12}, C, D, E, niacin, and folic acid.

The results showed that those subjects with the highest intake of vitamin C and folic acid were least likely to develop cataracts.

(*American Journal of Clinical Nutrition*, 6:435, 1987)

A Word About Folic Acid

The incidence of cancer could be greatly reduced if more people ate diets rich in folic acid.

Also, a rich supply of folic acid before and during pregnancy could greatly reduce the incidence of spina bifida, a serious health defect.

Imagine, an amount of folic acid small enough to fit on the end of your fingertip could help prevent cancer or, if you are a woman, help protect against giving birth to a child with spina bifida!

Where Can I Get Folic Acid?

Eat green leafy vegetables, Brewer's Yeast, liver, split peas, barley and brown rice.

You'll find folic acid in your multiple vitamin/mineral formula. 400 micrograms is the highest dose that can be sold without a prescription because higher doses can mask the symptoms of anemia. If you take the 400 micrograms in a multiple formula, it should be enough.

Seldom Supplemented Vitamin K May be More Important Than Thought

We rarely even think about vitamin K and never see it in a vitamin formula because it's rarely thought of as being deficient. But now it appears that vitamin K may lead to a better understanding of the aging process.

Vitamin K is found in leafy green vegetables. It helps the body manufacture a newly discovered amino acid called gamma-carboxyglutamic acid (GCA).

GCA has been found in 60 proteins in the lungs, liver, teeth, kidneys, and reproductive organs. Without enough vitamin K, those proteins either malfunction or cannot be manufactured at all.

This may be particularly important for the elderly because they suffer minor vitamin K deficiencies which could leave them vulnerable to illness.

Researchers estimate that most people need about 50 micrograms of vitamin K a day. You can get this from your diet if you eat some fresh broccoli, cabbage, spinach, Brussel's sprouts or other greens every day.

At his time, supplements do not appear to be necessary as long as dietary vegetable supplementation is part of your food.

Once again, grandma was right. Eat fresh, leafy greens every day to keep regular and live longer!

Senile Dementia? Maybe it's a Vitamin Deficiency

Perhaps 50 percent of the people said to be suffering from senile dementia (Alzheimer's disease) may actually have some other cause for mental deterioration.

That other cause — if discovered and treated — may result in a cure!

According to *American Family Physician* (36, No. 5:196, 1987), one of the hidden causes for a progressive difficulty in remembering can be overtreatment with diuretic medication (water pills). This can cause vitamin drainage which, in turn, can cause symptoms that seem as hopeless as Alzheimer's.

Another often overlooked cause is failure of the thyroid gland to release thyroid hormones. If recognized, this responds very quickly to prescriptions for thyroid extract tablets by mouth.

Astonishingly enough, a deficiency of vitamin B^{12} can also cause symptoms which are so close to that of Alzheimer's disease that they are often mistaken for that disease.

Normally, we get enough of the vitamin B^{12} from food. But, some people who eat very little animal food, and especially those who have had a lot of stomach trouble, lose their ability to absorb the vitamin as they grow older. The deficiency is not difficult to recognize in young people, but the focus is lost as people grow older and its effects become less typical and more easily confused with senile dementia.

If diagnosed soon enough, mental deterioration due to this lack responds to direct treatment with supplemental vitamin B^{12}. Many people protect themselves against a deficiency by taking up to 1,000 milligrams of B^{12} a day. You can get it at the health food store or drug store, or it may be included in your multi-vitamin/mineral formula.

To minimize the possibility of overlooking a reversible cause of dementia, elderly persons with memory failure should be seen as soon as possible by a physician specializing in geriatrics.

6

MINERALS

As with all vitamins, all minerals are essential to maintaining life and health. But, in the context of this book, a few minerals are more involved in youth restoration than others.

Toxicity of free radicals is thought to be a major factor in degenerative diseases and aging and those minerals which also act as antioxidants are essential for optimal health and lifespan.

Molybdenum

This mineral is a newcomer to the supplement scene. It is a trace mineral found in all tissues in the body and is required for the activity of several enzyme systems.

Compounds of molybdenum are rare. In nature, this element is hard to find in the Earth's crust and, in an area in China where it cannot be found in the soil, this scarcity has been associated with the world's highest incidence of esophageal cancer.

The mystery of its scarcity in the soil and its presence in all of our tissues has led to the postulate that life on earth did not begin on this planet but on some other planet with more abundant molybdenum in the environment!

This strange, scarce mineral may be an agent which works in the form of an activated enzyme to detoxify sulfites. It may also be a powerful antioxidant.

(*Proceedings of the National Academy of Sciences,* 78:6858, 1931)

We don't know enough about this nutrient.

The National Research Council recommends, as a safe and adequate daily ration, .15 to .5 milligrams for adults.

You'll have to read the label of your multi-mineral tablet or capsule to see if molybdenum is included. It should not be taken alone but in combination with other nutrients.

NOTE: People who suffer from gout or have high uric acid levels should consult with their physician before taking molybdenum. It can increase the levels of uric acid.

Manganese

Because it sounds like magnesium, manganese is frequently overlooked in mineral formulas.

It is required by the body in minute amounts, believed to be between 3 and 9 milligrams daily, but because it activates a number of enzyme reactions in the body, its absence can have far-reaching biochemical ramifications.

It is an element of the Glucose Tolerance Factor, the biological compound in our bodies which helps to regulate the metabolism of sugars and our energy supplies.

Managese also plays a role in regulating blood cholesterol levels and in maintaining the health of your heart.

Dr. Benjamin Frank, M.D., an authority on aging as it relates to nucleic acid functions in the cells, theorizes that a decline in cell energy transmission, affected by manganese deficiency, can result in several of the symptoms we associate with aging.

A good multi-mineral formula will contain some manganese. You will have to read the label carefully even if you have to carry a magnifying glass with you because the print is so small. If you eat a lot of whole grains and raw nuts and seeds, you may not need to take it as a supplement although the small amounts found in most formulas will only be a help. The change in the food supply from the kinds of foods our forefathers ate to the processed foods we eat today has produced many of the degenerative signals we see around us.

Other Reasons for Boning Up on Manganese

It may be an important factor in preventing osteoporosis and in fighting cell and tissue damage caused by a number of environmental insults.

For example:

Biologist Paul Saltman of the University of California at San Diego (UCSD) in La Jolla became interested in the importance of this trace mineral after meeting the physician taking care of basketball-superstar Bill Walton. Walton was constantly plagued by broken bones, many of which were difficult to heal.

When Walton's blood was analyzed, it was discovered that he had half the normal levels of zinc and copper but lots of calcium and *no* manganese.

Rats on a low-manganese diet develop porous bones.

Walton started taking mineral supplements and was back playing basketball in six weeks.

If you don't think that being able to build new bone and repairing existing bone structure doesn't play a part in the enjoyment of life, then you've never had a cast on your leg or arm.

(*Science News*, Sept. 27, 1986, Vol. 130, No. 13)

Chromium and Selenium, Two Key Minerals to Maintaining Youth

Selenium is found in adequate quantities in some areas but vast areas of the United States are deficient in this mineral.

And, if it's not in the soil it can't be found in the food grown on that soil.

Selenium helps to protect against the heavy metals cadmium and mercury. Mercury pollution is a growing health problem and cadmium (smoke and industrial waste) is a cause of hypertension.

Selenium helps prevent heredity changes involved in aging and in causing cancer. Areas which are low in selenium have higher cancer rates than areas which are normal in selenium content.

Selenium is an antioxidant which helps slow down the aging process which occurs in cells.

So you don't die as soon, and look far younger than your parents when they were the same age. In other words, adequate selenium intake will probably help to keep people younger and healthier.

Chromium

Is the shiny plating on your automobile bumper, and is also important for maintaining health.

It is involved in the metabolism of glucose and in the immune response to infection.

The sand rat, when fed the usual rat diet (which is better nutritionally than most human diets), develops diabetes. But, if returned to his natural habitat, he recovers from the disease.

How does this happen?

The sand rat seeks out and eats a plant called the desert saltbush which is rich in trivalent chromium, and when the rat gets enough chromium, his deficiency-induced diabetes is cured.

We know today that insulin is not effective without chromium being present in the body. In our country, chromium deficiency is common because food processing removes chromium from the foods which normally would supply it.

Chromium is most effective in an organic form called chromium picolinate. It consists of trivalent chromium, two niacin molecules, and the amino acids cystine, glycine and glutamic acid.

Foods which should provide chromium are liver, beef, beets, mushrooms, whole wheat, molasses and black pepper.

But supplementation is for insurance!

Humans are born with the highest percentage per body weight of chromium they will ever have.

With age, the proportion of chromium in the body decreases. Older people are among the groups that tend to exhibit symptoms of chromium deficiency. But, even with sophisticated equipment it's hard to detect.

How Much Should I Take?

For those interested in supplemental tablet forms, normal maintenance should be about 200 micrograms a day.

Chromium plays an integral part in human metabolism. You can chrome-plate your health for optimal performance and longevity. And, don't be surprised if you find yourself more energetic than you've ever been!

Other Minerals, Uses and Benefits

Calcium helps muscle tone, nerves, irritability and blood clotting. The supply of calcium can be dangerously low in the elderly. It is essential for bones and teeth and for preventing osteoporosis.

The National Institute of Health recommends 1,000 to 1,500 milligrams daily. You can get this amount from supplements or from milk and milk products, green leafy vegetables, citrus fruits, peas and beans.

Phosphorus is important for every tissue in the body. It is usually not necessary to supplement because it is found in such a wide variety of foods that a deficiency is an unusual event. In fact, due to the enormous consumption of phosphorous-containing carbonated soft drinks, excess phosphorous, which can leach calcium from the bones, might be a problem.

Potassium helps to regulate the balance and volume of body fluids. It is abundant in almost all foods, both plant and animal.

Iron transports and uses oxygen. Iron deficiency can be found in vegetarians, women with menstrual difficulties and people with metabolic disturbances. The RDA is 10 milligrams for men and 18 milligrams for women. Iron can be supplemented or obtained from liver, meat, eggs, fish, green leafy vegetables, legumes, prunes, whole grain cereal and iron-enriched flour.

Copper helps store and release iron for the red blood cells. It may be obtained from organ meats, shellfish, nuts and dried legumes.

Iodine controls the thyroid gland and prevents goiter. Foods from the sea and seaweeds are the best source outside of supplements.

Cobalt is bonded to vitamin B^{12} and serves as an essential element. It occurs only in trace amounts in plants and must be obtained either from animal foods or by supplementation.

Minerals and Longevity

Chromium picolinate

Protective against cardiovascular disease and high blood pressure.

(*American Journal of Clinical Nutrition,* 34:2670, 1981)

Copper

Protects cells and tissues against oxidative damage. It helps to prevent peroxidation (rancidity) of polyunsaturated fatty acids and maintains the integrity of cell membranes.

(*American Review of Respiratory Disease*, 126:3165, 1982)

Best when taken in a well-balanced vitamin/mineral formula. One such formula incorporates:

Copper	2 to 3 milligrams
Zinc	15 to 30 milligrams
Selenium	200 micrograms
Molybdenum	50 micrograms

Plus other vitamins and minerals.

(NOTE: Copper supplements should not be taken by persons suffering from Wilson's disease.)

Iron

Is involved in the structure of certain antioxidants like catalase, peroxidase and iron superoxide dismutase. The latter is found in bacteria.

It also stimulates resistance to infection.

(*Journal of Infectious Diseases*, 131:44, 1975)

Iron boosts physical performance of many kinds even when there is no anemia to cause muscle weakness and decreased exercise tolerance.

(*British Journal of Hematology*, 41:365, 1979)

Zinc

Essential to the development and maintenance of a healthy immune system and absolutely necessary for cell-mediated immunity.

(*Annual Review of Nutrition*, 2:151, 1982)

Zinc is required for the maintenance of our powers of taste, smell and vision. If there is a deficiency, we will not enjoy eating as much as we did when we were younger. Zinc supplementation can restore the senses and bring enjoyment back to the table!

(*Annals of Internal Medicine*, 99:227, 1983)

Also is able to increase the speed of wound healing.

(*Annals of Surgery*, 165:432, 1967)

Increases male potency and sex drive.

(*Nutrition Today*, Mar./Apr., 1981)

7

EXERCISE, LONGEVITY AND NUTRITION

AIDS is one of the most frightening diseases to afflict mankind. Out of approximately 57,000 cases (June, 1993) there were approximately 31,000 deaths. But, when compared to the statistics associated with cancer, these figures pale! In 1993, in the United States alone, approximately 980,000 new cases were reported with 550,000 deaths attributed to the disease.

AIDS and cancer have one thing in common besides fatalities. Both result from defects in the functioning of the immune system.

Cancer is a generic term for over 100 different diseases. It usually refers to a malignant tumor which arises from an abnormal and uncontrolled division of cells which then invade and destroy surrounding tissues. The spread of cancer cells throughout the body is called *metastasis,* and may occur via the bloodstream or the lymphatic system where secondary tumors may be set up.

Although there is no certainty about the cause of cancers, the currently accepted theory involves a two-step process known as *initiation* and *promotion.*

Initiation is the rapid, irreversible consequence of damage to important cellular components such as DNA. DNA is the key to cellular reproduction and damage to it results in imperfect cells from the mother cell.

Promotion entails the rapid division of the imperfect cell which ultimately takes over the surrounding areas and leads to the cancerous condition.

For example, take the case of the actor Steve McQueen. When he was a young man he worked as a longshoreman and was exposed to large amounts of asbestos. As he breathed in this substance, it caused some of the cells in his lungs to change (initiation). As he was also a heavy smoker, the chemicals in the smoke acted to promote the change (mutation) of the damaged cells in his lungs. In his thirties he succumbed to a type of cancer known as *mesothelioma*.

There are some things we can do to avoid shortening our lives. Stopping smoking is one of them. Avoiding hazardous substances, when we can, is another. Cutting fat from the diet is still another way because fats are easy prey to free radicals.

It is the free radicals which attack cellular membranes which can lead to the initiation phase of cancer.

Excess fats are also able to suppress the body's immune system, but luckily the body can defend itself against the free radicals by using natural antioxidants such as superoxide dismutase and dietary antioxidants such as certain vitamins, minerals, and amino acids. The vitamins include vitamins A, B-complex, C, E, beta-carotene. The minerals can be chromium, zinc, selenium, iron, magnesium, copper, manganese, molybdenum and calcium. The amino acids include methionine and L-cysteine.

By manipulating your diet you can help prevent the initiation phase. The American Cancer Society has issued a set of guidelines based on the best currently available research on cancer prevention.

1. Add cruciferous vegetables to your diet. These include cabbage, broccoli, Brussel's sprouts, cauliflower.
2. Increase vitamin A/beta-carotene containing foods.
3. Increase your intake of dietary fiber.
4. Increase your intake of vitamin C containing foods.
5. Reduce body fat levels through dieting and exercise.
6. Reduce total fat intake.
7. Avoid smoked, salt-cured or nitrate-cured foods.
8. Don't smoke.
9. Minimize alcohol consumption.
10. Cut down exposure to the sun.

How Can Exercise Help Me Live Longer?

There are a number of ways exercise helps you. One way is its effects on the fatty cholesterol particles in the blood.

Fats in the blood are called triglycerides, the same type of fat found under the skin. Fats are not soluble in water and not soluble in our waterways we call the bloodstream so, in order to travel around the body, they are attached to a blood protein. That's when they are called a lipoprotein and are able to move around the system.

When you have your cholesterol measured, you usually get a total amount which is for the percent of cholesterol in your blood. But it doesn't tell you about the size of the particles and the size is important to the risk of cardiovascular problems.

The smallest lipoproteins are dense and contain less fat. These are called HDL (high-density-lipoproteins). They protect against the development of fatty cholesterol deposits in the arteries which lead to arteriosclerosis and related diseases which certainly shorten life.

The medium sized lipoproteins contain more fat and are called LDL (low-density-lipoproteins). These are the problem-causing particles that tend to deposit in the walls of arteries and cause blockages, heart attacks, strokes and other problems.

Then there are very large lipoproteins with lots of fats. They have a very low density and are called LDL for obvious reasons. The main function of these is to transport fat through the bloodstream.

When you go for a check-up, ask for the percentages of all of these fractions.

It is desirable to have lots of HDL cholesterol and very little of the LDL cholesterol.

Studies show that exercise tends to increase the HDL cholesterol and lower the triglycerides and LDL cholesterol.

This is exactly what you want to do to decrease your risk of cardiovascular disease and extend your lifespan.

Exercise and Blood Clotting

Although there are many benefits to exercise and many books have been written about increasing lung capacity and heart strength, etc., this book is concerned with longevity.

A major factor in heart attacks and strokes is the formation of a blood clot. A clot in a coronary artery which is already partially blocked with fatty cholesterol deposits can be fatal. A clot which forms in a vein in the leg may dislodge and go to the lungs, resulting in a pulmonary embolism which may be sudden death.

Inactivity promotes the formation of blood clots.

In the past years it has been found that injecting certain enzymes into the blood of patients having an acute heart attack will dissolve the clot and may protect the heart muscle from infarction. One of the best of the enzymes is a substance called tissue plasminogen activator (TPA). It helps to dissolve the strands of fibrin that make a clot harden.

Physical activity stimulates the release of TPA into the circulation.

In addition, exercise helps to decrease obesity. Fat people manufacture less TPA than lean people do. Inactivity discourages TPA production. Bed rest is notorious as a factor in causing clots in the leg.

How Much Physical Activity Is Needed?

As little as five minutes of strenuous exercise may increase this clot prevention through TPA for two hours. This is a strong argument for people who work sitting down to get up and do some form of exercise several times a day. Even several short walks during the day will significantly improve the TPA activity. Since many heart attacks occur in the early morning hours, a walk in the morning to help decrease the tendency to early-morning-clotting could be a life saver.

Another factor involved in blood clotting is the thickness of the blood. The test for thickness is done by measuring the percent of the blood volume that is liquid and the percent that is composed of blood cells. The test for this is the hematocrit. The more you exercise, the more the blood moves smoothly through the vessels. Inactive people have blood that is more sluggish.

Fish oil from eating fatty fish or taking fish oil capsules, helps to make the blood less inclined to clot. So, a reasonable exercise program, eating fish or taking fish oil capsules and one aspirin tablet every other day can offer a longer and happier life!

8

WHY MUST WE WAIT?

Headline: February 15, 1988. "Privileged Breakthrough Information — Miracle Cancer Protection Coming."

Safe compounds derived from vegetables may prevent many different forms of cancer. Used as dietary supplements or food additives, they could save millions of lives each year.

Cancer prevention, rather than treatment, may be the best hope for saving lives.

(And it goes on and on about the inability of other techniques — cutting, radiation, hormones etc. to stem the tide of cancer deaths.)

New Hope: PROTEASE INHIBITORS — substances found in chick-peas soybeans, potatoes and other vegetables — can halt cancer development at an early stage.

They block the action of specific proteases and seem to be able to stop cells from turning malignant.

Animal tests show that they are more resistant to colon, liver, and oral cancer.

Then. . . we are told that tests on humans have begun.

What Do We Do Till Then?

We take a lesson from a book written by Jay M. Davis, M.D., Ph.D., called *Until A Cure Comes.*

Dr. Davis is in favor of using what he calls, "inexpensive substances which can provide a powerful shield against cancer."

Selenium

Selenium offers protection against cancer of the breast, skin, colon, lung, liver, leukemia. In order to be effective, a certain minimum dose is needed. The longer you supplement the better.

Mechanism of Action

According to the doctor, the consensus is that selenium exerts its protective effect via the enzyme glutathione peroxidase. This compound destroys peroxides which are highly active compounds produced during metabolism.

(Most of you have put hydrogen peroxide on a cut at one time or another and have seen it merrily bubbling away. When it bubbles inside the body it creates havoc and cellular destruction.)

The peroxides are capable of damaging the DNA, the material that genes are made of, and thus big suspects in the cause of cancer.

However, a new concept of selenium's action in the body is exciting another look. It appears that selenium is also capable of improving the immune system's action against cancer cells.

Dietary sources of selenium are typically listed as organ meats, sea food and cereal grains but there's not a lot of selenium involved in most diets.

What Should I Take?

According to what I read, a top of 300 micrograms a day of the organic form of selenium (Selenomethionine).

Selenium and Other Nutrients

Dr. Davis also writes about selenium and vitamin A supplementation as protective to the body, offering results better than if either is used alone.

He also goes into the use of beta-carotene and its ability to destroy free radicals, and the use of antioxidants like vitamin C and vitamin E.

The book finishes with the doctor's own protective supplemental program:

1. *Selenium* 300 micrograms (although the RDA is 50 to 200 micrograms)
2. *Vitamin E* 400 I.U.
3. *B-carotene* 15 to 30 milligrams daily
4. *Vitamin A* 10,000 I.U. daily
5. *Vitamin C* 500 mg daily

What is most important about this book is that it is written by an M.D. and it carefully traces medically established criteria to come up with conclusions that the health food industry has hinted at for a number of years:

Supplements Can Help You to Avoid Certain Cancers.

(The book, *Until a Cure Comes,* was printed by Miller Press, 1840 Myrtle Ave., Eureka, CA 95501)

The Doctor Rinse Formula. . . Free To Anyone Who Wants It!

Dr. Jacobus Rinse was born in Holland and has a doctorate in physical chemistry. When he was 51 he had his first heart attack and was told he had, at most, ten years to live.

Six years later he suffered his second severe heart attack, even though he was now taking garlic, vitamin C and vitamin E and avoiding strenuous exercise.

With six of his ten years gone, he figured that he needed all of the remaining four years to come up with some concept that could prolong his life.

He is, at the time of this writing, 89 years old and GOING STRONG!

What Did He Do?

He used his brains. Certain scientific tests done on animals suggested that lecithin could actually dissolve cholesterol. In addition, safflower oil was shown to contain factors which could work with lecithin to liquify cholesterol. He thought it was entirely possible that a combination of the two could conquer atherosclerosis and clear clogged arteries.

Along with the other supplements, he began to take one tablespoon of lecithin and one tablespoon of safflower oil every day.

His angina pains ceased and his pulse rate began to decrease. After a short period of time he began to feel much better.

He is certainly a representative of "the Unstoppables," men and women who came out of disease younger than when they went in.

He then thought out the supplements the body needed and devised a mixture that would supply them.

He didn't make a dime from the formula but gave it out freely to anyone who wanted to use it. Although some companies have put the Dr. Rinse formula on the market and sell it to those who don't want to take the trouble to make it for themselves, here is the mixture that was and is being used by Dr. Rinse today.

The Dr. Rinse Formula

A two-week supply will require the following:

- 7 tablespoons of lecithin granules
- 6 tablespoons of raw wheat germ
- 6 tablespoons debittered brewer's yeast in powder or flake form
- 6 tablespoons of sunflower seeds
- 6 teaspoons bonemeal in powder or tablet form
- 6 vitamin C tablets of 500 milligrams each
- 6 vitamin E tablets of 200 I.U. each

Crush the seeds and the tablets in a blender until finely ground, then mix all the rest of the ingredients together.

Store in a well-closed jar in the refrigerator.

Take 1 or 2 tablespoons daily.

Mix it with honey if you want to, or into your oatmeal at breakfast time.

It's Not What You Eat But What You Can Digest — The Role of Enzymes and Raw Food

Disease prevention can depend on digestive enzymes. According to Dr. Edward Howell, author of *Food Enzymes for Health and Longevity*, Omangod Press, Conn., 1980, "If experiments on animals held true for humans, it could mean that people could extend their lifespans by 20 or more years — just by maintaining proper enzyme levels."

Did you ever stop to think of the food situation before fire became man's best friend? Everything was eaten as is — raw, if it was animal food, or natural, if it was vegetable food.

And mankind flourished and survived under the worst conditions and hardships.

Then, one sloppy caveman dropped his share of bear meat into the newly-discovered fire and discovered "cooking." Because of that one sloppy moment, cooked food was in and enzymes were out!

Food cooked above 118 degrees F. destroys all of the natural enzymes. That's when the body has to supply digestive enzymes from the salivary glands, pancreas, stomach, and intestines. Protease, lipase, amylase must be released to break down protein, carbohydrates, and fats into a form the body can utilize.

As we age, the efficiency of the digestive system lessens and less and less of the nutrient value of the food we eat is absorbed. Many scientists believe that this situation is one of the main causes of allergies and disease.

When a study of the pancreas of Filipinos and Malay people was made by Professor Schaefer of the Mayo Foundation, it was found that the organ was 25 to 50 percent heavier than that of Occidentals. The cause of this weight difference was ascribed to the fact that they depended on cooked rice as their staple food, eating it three times a day.

Professor Jackson of the Department of Anatomy, University of Minnesota, has shown that an 80 percent cooked food diet fed to laboratory animals for 155 days resulted in an increased pancreatic weight of 20 to 30 percent.

A cooked food diet strains the digestive system, making it work harder than it would have to if the diet were composed of raw food. Also, cooked food tends to travel through the digestive tract more slowly than raw food, with the result that it tends to ferment and liberates gas and toxic material. This can cause gas, heartburn, headaches and many more serious conditions. The recent information blitz about fiber and the benefits which can accrue when you add more fiber to the diet is really a plea for adding raw foods to what you eat. Only bulky, fiber-type raw food will exercise the intestines in an adequate manner, cleaning out small, pain-causing, disease-causing particles that collect in the pockets and the elbows of your intestines.

The emphasis on grains, raw fruit and vegetables, bran, etc. helps to keep the digestive tract free from putrefaction and the problems of autointoxication.

Digestive problems have been described in detail for at least the last 500 years. Among the most common are those connected with incomplete digestion. Bad breath, bloat, skin problems, muscle wasting, diminished immunity to disease, delayed wound healing, anemia, poor bowel function, depression, allergies, irritable bowel syndrome, colitis, and diverticulitis.

No Energy?

Digestion is the first step in the conversion of food into the energy you have to have to stay alive. Everything you need to run your body, except for oxygen, has to go through the digestive tract.

According to Time-Life Books, about 90,000 pounds of food and 55,000 quarts of fluid pass through our digestive tract in a lifetime.

In the most unromantic way, we are a conveyor belt. Food goes in one end, is treated with chemicals so the nutrients can be separated from the waste material, the nutrients are absorbed and the waste material goes out the other end.

The enzymes found in food help us to digest them. But living enzymes are found only in raw food. Foods like cabbage, carrots, tomatoes, cucumbers, endives, avocadoes, mangoes, bananas, apples, oranges, grapefruits, lemons, papayas, pineapple, figs, and sprouts. Lactic acid foods such as yogurt and kefir, sauerkraut and sour bread.

What Do Enzymes From Food Have To Do With Living Longer?

Besides sparing you all of the unpleasant symptoms, like the way you feel after a heavy meal, enzymes from raw foods will spare the body's enzyme reserve, leaving it intact for other important metabolic functions such as helping the body heal itself from disease. Metabolic enzymes keep your body running, providing the means for many biochemical reactions involved with metabolism. They repair damage and decay in addition to healing.

Enzymes are part of the immune system. When the white blood cells have engulfed an invading bacteria, it is the enzymes that actually dissolve them.

If You Don't Make Enzymes, Take Them!

Most health food stores and drug stores carry digestive and other enzymes. If there is a case of chronic or acute pancreatic insufficiency (ask your health professional), the Mayo clinic has demonstrated that 5NF pancreatin is useful in the digestion and absorption of both protein and fats.

A light colored stool is usually indicative of a lack of bile. Beet leaf juice powder is a good choice if this is your complaint. Check with your doctor of course.

Bile production naturally needs vitamin C, magnesium, copper, and the amino acid taurine in adequate amounts.

Some enzyme formulas contain papain from papaya and bromelain from the pineapple, plus digestive enzymes from animal sources. They should be taken with meals to facilitate digestion.

Apple pectin tablets are available to help emulsify and digest fats.

Supplements should be used to help your system normalize, take the strain away for a while — about 2 to 3 months. After that start to taper them off. Your body will welcome the change if you have added a lot of raw foods to your diet.

Additional Support for Raw Foods

The book, *The Hippocrates Diet and Health Program,* by Ann Wigmore, Avery Publishing Group, Inc., 1984, is a fascinating study of how what we eat affects our health.

Although her entire book is germane to this book and other books devoted to health, the particular idea she expounds that each meal makes deposits into your enzyme account is both expressive and accurate.

As to healing, enzymes break down excess fat to be eliminated in weight loss. You have to agree that if you are carrying around too much extra fat you are shortening your lifespan.

Many obese individuals have decreased levels of fat-splitting enzymes.

So, if it's weight loss you're after, or reversal of any other form of deposit in the body such as calcium in arthritis, excess protein in tumors, or cholesterol in atherosclerosis, only enzymes can break them up and eliminate them.

Likewise, if you are in the need of a few more pounds, stronger teeth or bones, sharper eyesight, or stronger muscles, enzymes can help you.

Just to include plenty of high-quality protein, minerals and vitamins in the diet will not do. Metabolic enzymes are also required to build these nutrients into blood, bones, nerves, organs, and tissues.

As we age, our enzyme workers desert us unless we take steps to stop the one-way flow out of the body. We need both metabolic and digestive enzymes. If we don't supply them, the body will rob metabolic enzymes to do digestive enzyme jobs. Food enzymes have to be ingested so they can do some of the job.

Understanding Nature and Digestion

A python swallows a pig whole.

But, not until the final stages do the snake's own enzymes have to function. Up until then, all of the digestive processes have come from the pig itself.

If we eat pork, all the digestion must come from our own enzymes.

Chickens and other birds have a crop, a food enzyme stomach, which holds the seeds and grains the bird eats for up to twelve hours. During that time the seeds begin to sprout and this sprouting starts the predigestion of the proteins, fats and starches in the food.

We, however, have to digest food from scratch.

If you have a meal of pizza, a cola, a couple of twinkies and a glass of pasteurized milk, you have committed your stomach to 4 hours of unending work.

But, if that meal consists of salad greens and tomatoes with lemon dressing, whole grain wheat bread, and raw fruit with herbal tea, there will be sufficient pre-digestion in the stomach to ease the burden on your own organs.

Natural enzyme aids, in addition to what we spoke about earlier, include:

- Wheatgrass juice, the chlorophyll extract of 7-day-old wheat plants which contain an abundance of magnesium, enzymes, chlorophyll, vitamins and minerals
- Green drinks from sprouts, greens, vegetables, plus a little sauerkraut juice to taste
- Lemon juice
- Carrot juice, high in vitamin A and beta-carotene
- Beet juice. Take small quantities and sip slowly
- Apple juice, or fresh cider

Vitamins and Cancer

Two studies, one on lung cancer and vitamins and the other on cervical cancer and vitamins, asks — what connection do vitamin levels have with cancer?

The first study involved researchers from Louisiana State University Medical School in New Orleans. They found significantly lower levels of vitamins E and C in patients suffering from cancer of the lung when compared to a group of healthy control subjects. Although low levels of vitamin A were associated with lung cancer in earlier testings, the new study indicated that vitamins E and C may be as important as vitamin A or even more important.

(*American Journal of Clinical Nutrition*, April, 1985)

The second study was done at the University of Alabama in Birmingham. It was found that 67 percent of people with cervical cancer had at least one abnormal vitamin value while 18 percent had three or more low values.

Folic acid, beta-carotene, and vitamin C levels were the nutrients most usually found at low levels.

(*American Journal of Obstetrics and Gynecology*, March, 1985)

Although there is so much continuing research about nutrition and disease, there is still reluctance in the medical community to confirm the connection. There may be no way to obtain the nutrient level necessary to ward off disease or implement healing from a disease by means of the diet alone. Supplementation *and* a healthful diet however, will increase the levels of vitamins and minerals to the point where our body is capable of healing itself and preventing the unwelcome intrusion of invading pathogens.

9

MORE ACTION AGAINST DISEASE

An extract from the common egg is offering new hope for a variety of health problems and agonizing, life-shortening diseases, including the immune problems associated with AIDS, herpes, aging, and Epstein-Barr virus (CFS).

It is a special form of egg lecithin known as 7-2-1, because of its composition of about 7 parts neutral lipids, 2 parts of phosphatidyl choline, and 1 part phosphatidyl ethanolamine.

Its use as a possible adjunctive treatment against AIDS was first publicized in the AIDS Treatment News (ATN) on April 1986 by the medical writer John S. James. It reported the case of an AIDS victim who was treated at the Weizmann Institute of Science in Israel, and who — according to his own accounts — recovered from the symptoms.

(Current medical science reports show that investigations into the possible use of the 7-2-1 formula are ongoing at a medical college in N.Y.)

On the immunity front, there are some findings that egg-derived lecithin may have immune-enhancing properties that have not been known or investigated in the past. Lecithin does play a number of roles in maintaining health. (We've already written about its ability to break down fat and cholesterol deposits and its helping to reverse conditions such as arteriosclerosis and atherosclerosis, which substantially reduces the chances of heart attack and stroke.)

Lecithin, as a source of choline and a precursor of acetylcholine, has been linked with such conditions as Parkinson's disease, learning difficulties and memory loss, and supplementation can be helpful in a number of these cases.

However, the role of lecithin and immune function has not been widely known because very few reports have been written and circulated in the medical community.

There were only four published reports which tried lecithin on viral hepatitis with reasonable success. The helpful nature of the lecithin was attributed to the phosphatidyl choline content.

Another research paper dealt with cell membrane fluidity. Membranes are made from proteins, cholesterols and phospholipids. Fluidity is the degree to which the protein circulates. The fluidity decreases when cholesterol increases as we age, making the cell membrane easier to attack. When healthy, the membrane serves as a barrier against invasion by bacteria, yeasts, and viruses. It also permits the entrance of essential nutrients into the cell.

The work done at the Weizman Institute showed that aging cells became "stiff" and less resistant to invasion. They began to look for a means of reversing the stiffness and restoring the membrane fluidity. Since cell membranes are largely made of lecithin, and egg lecithin is similar to the lecithin in human tissue — even more similar than the lecithin from soy — it was chosen for investigation.

The chief investigator, Dr. Meier Shinitzky, found that one form of egg lecithin was as much as ten times more effective as a membrane fluidizer than any other form. It not only made the membrane less stiff, but it also aided the removal of cholesterol from the membrane, helping to reverse the aging process.

Human studies on elderly people showed an increased ability to fight off infection. Laboratory tests also showed that the 7-2-1 compound was able to neutralize viruses in the test tube. Tests are now being done to see if the same results could neutralize viruses in humans. If it works, the implications for viral conditions, including AIDS could be far-reaching.

10

AMINO ACIDS PLUS LONGER LIFE

What Are Amino Acids?

They are organic compounds made of carbon, hydrogen, oxygen and nitrogen (as differentiated from fats and carbohydrates which are made up of carbon, hydrogen and oxygen alone) and combinations of these organic compounds go to make up all proteins.

These combinations can range from just a few to many thousands, all arranged in a chain.

All protein foods are composed of amino acids. The digestive system breaks them down into individual acids and then reassembles them into the arrangement the body needs.

Different tissues need different arrangements.

Growing muscle, for example, needs to assemble branched chain amino acids for the most part. They are called leucine, isoleucine and valine. Bodybuilders frequently take loads of these amino acids in a free form (not bound to other amino acids or to proteins) to help them attain larger muscle mass.

Much of the research on amino acids indicates that there is a good deal of potential benefit from them.

Where Can I Get Them?

Health food stores and drug stores usually stock a variety of amino acids. But you should know more about them before you take them.

Arginine and Ornithine

It is claimed that arginine can make the body burn fat while building muscle, even if you're doing nothing more than watching TV on your couch. In fact, arginine does have a definite stimulating effect on human growth hormone, which, in turn, can do a number of fantastic things.

That does not mean you should pop great quantities of this amino acid because not everything is known about its use when taken alone. When we take in amino acids in the normal manner, they are usually in combinations.

It has been shown that oral intake of arginine, especially in combination with lysine, caused the release of the biologically active growth hormone.

In this testing, 1200 milligrams of arginine were given with 1200 milligrams of lysine.

But the study did not show whether the release of growth hormone did build muscle or burn fat. . . just that it did release the hormone and that could be the result!

(*Current Medical Research and Opinion*, 7:475, 1981)

Arginine does speed the healing of wounds. That may be a result of that hormone release.

(*Surgery*, August 1978, p.224)

Arginine stimulates the immune system. It does this by stimulating the thymus gland and related thymic processes.

(*Journal of Parenteral and Enteral Nutrition*, 4:446, 1980)

Arginine inhibits the growth of various tumors in laboratory animals, probably by virtue of its immune system stimulation.

(*Journal of Parenteral and Enteral Nutrition*, 4:446, 1980)

Natural sources of arginine include raw cereals, various nuts, and — chocolate lovers —your favorite chocolate!

Since definitive studies have not been done, ask your doctor or coach about dosage.

Growth hormone, from the pituitary gland, decreases in production after the age of thirty. This may be the reason that arginine has been effective in general cases of debility where the immune system has been weakened. By toning the system, arginine (sometimes with ornithine) can reduce recovery time drastically.

Its anti-cancer therapeutic use can be accentuated by additional supplementation of free radical fighters such as vitamins A,

E, C, B^1, and B^5, as well as the minerals selenium and zinc and the amino acid L-cysteine.

DID YOU KNOW THAT CHICKEN SOUP IS A NATURAL SOURCE OF BOTH ARGININE AND ORNITHINE?

Your mother knew it. It strengthens the body and helps to end disease.

Arginine also plays a vital role in the urea cycle, an important metabolic process that detoxifies ammonia.

CAUTION: This amino acid supplement is not for youngsters. In the young it can cause bone damage.

These growth-enhancing amino acids should not be confused with the growth hormones now being taken by some athletes. The growth hormones they use to stimulate muscle mass are actually steroids and should not be used by anyone unless prescribed by a physician for a disease.

But Can They Grow Hair?

L-cysteine can strengthen the skin, nails, and hair and for this reason is included in many of the "hair growth formulas" on the market.

But Will It Grow Hair?

I don't think so.

The hair-raising idea comes from the fact that certain wool producers have found that enriching their sheep's diet with this amino acid significantly increases wool production.

When dog owners heard about this, they added some L-cysteine to their dog food and found that their pets grew longer, more luxurious coats.

Unless you have a good head of hair, L-cysteine (taken with food) will do very little good, and possibly some harm if you are a diabetic. Large doses of L-cysteine may interfere with insulin. Also, when you take this amino acid, make sure that you take 2 or 3 times the amount of vitamin C along with it.

L-cysteine's main claim to fame, along with methionine and taurine, is that it contains the element sulfur. These three amino acids act as free radical deactivators, neutralizing certain toxins, and aiding protein synthesis.

(NOTE: All amino acids should be taken in the L- form. The label will list them as L-cysteine, L-methionine, L-taurine, L-arginine, L-tryptophan, etc. *The D- form should not be used.*)

According to John Mann, author of *Secrets of Life Extension,* L-cysteine is the most powerful of the three for detoxification. In nature it is found in the "smelly" foods such as cabbage, eggs, onions and garlic.

L-cysteine helps transport toxic heavy metals out of the body. It detoxifies acetaldehyde, a poison found in cigarette smoke and smog, and is a natural byproduct in alcohol metabolism. It also offers some protection against radiation.

L-cysteine is also a precursor of the free radical fighter glutathione, mentioned earlier in this book.

The following is a breakdown of the major areas of amino acid supplementation when used for therapeutic action. Many formulas found in health food and drug stores apply these combinations, or similar combinations with vitamins and minerals, along with exercise and diet, as alternative methods for controlling certain conditions.

Amino acids used in this manner bear more of a resemblance to drug therapy than supplement therapy and should be approached in a more cautious manner.

Therapeutic Uses for Amino Acids

Heavy Metal Detoxification

Methionine, cysteine, cystine
Histidine

Counteracting Free Radical Activity

Glutathione
Methionine

Assistance in Fatty Metabolism

Methionine
Taurine
Carnitine

Acceleration of Wound Healing

Arginine
Proline

Control of Viral Infection

Lysine

Thymus Gland Activity

Arginine

Enhanced Insulin Production/Glucose Tolerance Improvement

Arginine
Taurine
Cysteine

Immune System Enhancement

Glutathione

Brain Detoxification (of ammonia)

Glutamic Acid

Protection Against Radiation Effects

Histadine
Glutathione
Cysteine

Weight Control

Phenylalanine
Tryptophan
Valine
Methionine
Carnitine

Depression

Phenylalanine
Tryptophan
Tyrosine
Glutamic Acid

Insomnia

Tryptophan

Aging Process (skin)

Proline
Glutathione

Aging (in general)

All amino acids
Glutathione

Circulation

Carnitine
Taurine

Brain Fuel

Glutamine is converted to glutamic acid in the brain

Hair Health

Cysteine

Pain Control

Tryptophan
DLPA

NOTE: When purchasing amino acids, follow label directions.

PART II

CONCENTRATED "BETTER SEX" FOODS FOR WOMEN

11

CONCENTRATED "BETTER SEX" FOODS FOR WOMEN

Can what you eat help you to have a better sex life?

Can food and/or nutritional supplements influence your relationships?

Is there anything you can do to increase your sexual potency and your sexual enjoyment?

Do you understand the intimate relationship between food and sex?

The answer to questions one, two and three is YES!

If you don't know the answer to question four, this part has been written for YOU.

Not only can your choice of foods influence your good health and good sex by reducing the chance of diseases such as arteriosclerosis, diabetes and so on, but your choices of the types of nutritional supplements you take can actually promote a better sexual frame of mind.

Nutritional supplements, when you know which one does what, can promote energy, delay fatigue, promote a faster recovery for more and better sex, and can actually feed your brain the brain chemicals (neurotransmitters) to make you "feel sexier" and respond more powerfully than ever before.

Nutritional supplements can help you get rid of nasty fat, the flab that gets between you and good sex. Lean and hard promotes better sexual contact and makes for a more attractive you. Lean and hard even "feels" sexy.

Some nutritional supplements can play a dual role in helping you to help yourself to more and better sex play. L-phenylalanine, for example, can help you lose weight and stimulate more sexual pleasure at the same time. That's only one of the many "secrets" to be discovered here to give you the kind of sex life you deserve.

Another is L-carnitine, the fat burner that burns up excess fat in your bloodstream while building your energy levels to teenage heights.

If you're satisfied with your sex life, this section can make it even better.

If you're not satisfied, this section may make all the difference in the world!

A Sexy Body Needs Vitamins

You have to work at sex whether you like it or not. You have to treat your body with tender love and care if you want someone else to do the same.

Love and flab don't go together.

Hard and firm go with sex and love.

Food, vitamins and minerals can make the difference between satisfaction and "who cares."

Tissues, glands and organs must receive the kind of nourishment that makes them contribute to the kind of mood, feeling, energy level and behavior that calls for the kind of sex life you deserve.

Most women think they have sex problems when they really have nutrition problems. Nutrition problems are much easier to solve, and much cheaper to deal with than genuine sex problems.

Diet is important, and adequate vitamin supplementation makes up for some of the dietary insufficiencies and supports the body while it's making up for years of neglect.

You Need Vitamin A for Lubrication

Vitamin A keeps mucous membrane and your skin in good repair. Mucous membrane covers the throat, inside of the nose, the gastrointestinal tract, and the genital area. Mucous membrane must be kept moist in order to function at its best. Dry skin rubbing against skin is uncomfortable at best and painful at its worst. Dry skin can crack and bleed and certainly work against any kind of sexual contact. Dry skin is also more prone to bacterial invasion so keeping your skin and mucous membrane soft and beautiful instead of dry and scaly is of paramount importance for sex and health.

Vitamin A cannot be manufactured in the body and has to be gotten from the diet or from supplements. If there is a deficiency of vitamin A, your man can find his testicles shriveling and you can suffer shriveling of the ovaries, as shown in test cases with male and female laboratory animals. In males, sperm formation is cut down and in pregnant female rats, the fetus can be reabsorbed.

Lack of this important vitamin is believed to have a deleterious effect upon hormone production, particularly the sex hormones.

Vitamin A and vitamin E should be used together since a combination of the two increases the power of either one. Vitamin A is stored in the liver, kidneys, lungs and fatty tissue in the body.

The main sources of vitamin A in the diet are fish, liver, eggs, cheese and dairy products.

Beta-carotene is the vegetable form of vitamin A. It can be as useful or even more useful than vitamin A because it can never be harmful to the body. I bring this matter up because extremely high doses of vitamin A may be harmful if administered over a long period of time. I am referring to doses of 50,000 I.U. or more. Usually the use of vitamin A in amounts up to 25,000 I.U. daily will not cause any harm; however, beta-carotene can be used in any amount. The secret lies in the fact that beta-carotene is two molecules of vitamin A locked together. When it is locked, it has no vitamin A activity and no ill effects no matter how high the dosage normally used. When the body has a need for vitamin A it simply unlocks the molecule and releases the amount of vitamin A it needs.

Beta-carotene, in addition to its sexually explicit tasks, can also protect the body against toxins, radiation, free radicals and is a stimulant to the immune system.

Beta-carotene can be obtained from green leafy vegetables, broccoli, peas, sweet potatoes, yams, carrots, cantaloupes, peaches and apricots.

If you like herbs, it is found in parsley, dandelion, mint and alfalfa.

Vitamin B-Complex

This entire family of vitamins is water soluble which means they must be obtained daily, either from the diet or from the use of supplements. They are easily washed out of the body or lost during cooking in water. This is one reason that you should steam vegetables for a short period of time or else eat them raw. If you do cook them in water, save the water and drink it or use it as a gravy.

Vitamin B^1

Vitamin B^1 is essential to energy production and the metabolism of fats, carbohydrates and proteins. If you are deficient in this vitamin, you will have less energy for living and even less to spend on good sex.

Even if you take in a quantity of this vitamin but drink a lot of coffee or alcoholic beverages, or even if you drink a load of tea, you can destroy much of the vitamin B^1 in your body. Besides a lack of interest in sex you can also show the following symptoms: fatigue, apathy, slowed reflexes, constipation, indigestion and even a rapid pulse rate.

Best food sources include raw nuts and seeds like sunflower seeds, beans, asparagus, pineapple, yogurt, whole wheat, wheat germ, brown rice, whole grains, liver, lean meat, beans.

Herbs containing B^1 include mint, dandelion, parsley, fenugreek and bladderwick.

Most authorities believe that supplements, in varying strengths, are a good idea because its difficult to count on the food supply as a constant source of vitamins, vitamin B^1 included.

Vitamin B^2

Stress can create a temporary deficiency of this important vitamin and bad food can create a more permanent deficiency. B^2 is soluble in water so you have to get some every day from food or supplements.

A deficiency can rob the body of energy. No energy means no sex. B^2 is a part of the energy-producing metabolic process. If you're tired all the time and have any of the following deficiency signs, you may be having a B^2 problem:

- cracks at the corner of the mouth
- glossitis of the tongue
- burning, tearing eyes
- a fear of light
- slow wound healing (also a sign of a zinc deficiency)

Food sources of vitamin B^2 include milk, beef liver, green vegetables, raw nuts and seeds, wheat germ, brown rice, broccoli and asparagus. Herbs are alfalfa and parsley.

Vitamin B^3 (Niacin)

One of the wonder vitamins which can help you beat a cholesterol problem as well as a sex problem.

A chronic deficiency can cause a situation called pellagra (skin eruptions, mental problems, anorexia, bowel problems). Pellagra used to be a big problem in the southern part of the United States where corn only was the staple food. Corn is lacking vitamin B^3.

A niacin deficiency can hamper sex through the nervous system and through the digestive system. An abundance of niacin can greatly stimulate your enjoyment of sex. Niacin dilates the blood vessels, stimulating circulation and causing a "niacin flush" during sex. This can be very arousing to the female, even eliciting orgasm in cases where it has been an elusive prize.

Food sources of B^3 (niacin) are basically the same as B^2, plus chicken, fish, dates, raw almonds and yogurt.

If you take niacin as a supplement, watch out for the flush that will occur. It is not dangerous but can be scary if you don't expect it. In fact, chest, upper arms and head will turn red and you'll feel warm and tingly all over. This can be great fun during sexual encounters.

If you don't want the flush, try taking small doses, such as 50 mg. with meals, and gradually build up to a larger dose. Or, try to get a time-release tablet that dissolves over a period of time.

Cholesterol levels have been lowered with this vitamin and, of course, clearer blood vessels are great contributors to good sex.

Vitamin B^6

Also known as pyridoxine, B^6 is necessary for the metabolism of amino acids, and amino acids have a profound effect upon energy and sexual desire and performance. Vitamin B^6 decreases prolactin, a hormone that diminishes a women's sexual arousal.

Vitamin B^6 is involved in the production of neurotransmitters (brain chemicals) which are involved in orgasm. If you're on the "pill," it's possible that you are deficient in this very sexy vitamin. A lack of B^6 can cause a loss of sex drive.

Food sources include wheat germ, brown rice, whole grains, liver, eggs, raw nuts and seeds and molasses.

Pantothenic Acid

Another member of the B-complex family of vitamins and also closely involved in energy production. Pantothenic acid helps make the steroid hormones and the steroid hormones help make you better in bed. Pantothenic acid is also involved in the manufacture of acetylcholine, one of the more important neurotransmitters. In fact, acetylcholine is necessary for sexual arousal and some experts have said that large amounts improve sexual performance.

Food sources include liver, milk, eggs, whole grains, nuts, seeds, poultry, fish, broccoli, cabbage and cauliflower.

Biotin

Just a tiny amount is needed to keep you on an even keel, but the lack of this B-vitamin can cause a depressed state. That's the reason you'll find it in any good B-complex vitamin supplement.

If you eat cereals, vegetables, milk or liver, you'll get enough from the diet.

PABA

Para-aminobenzoic acid helps keep your hair, skin and bowels in good order. Certainly, all three are important to a good sex life.

Folic Acid

This vitamin is most lacking in American diets because it is so easily destroyed by our cooking methods and by stress. When it is deficient, it can be the cause of spontaneous abortion, fetal malformation, anemia or chromosomal damage.

Food sources include green leafy vegetables, broccoli, Brussels sprouts, asparagus, sprouts, raw nuts and seeds.

Choline

When people recommend lecithin as a cholesterol controlling agent, it is the choline content that makes it work. High blood pressure, kidney trouble, arteriosclerosis and diabetes have been linked to high cholesterol levels, and people suffering from any of these diseases are not as interested in sex as they could be. Therefore, a high choline intake in the form of lecithin (try 2 lecithin capsules, 1200 mg each with meals or better yet, take 1 tablet of Phos-Cal which is phosphatidyl choline 95 percent, with meals), is going to be of help to your sex life. Choline is a major part of the neurotransmitter acetylcholine which is said to take part in sexual arousal.

Food sources include eggs, meat, poultry, fish, soybeans, whole grains and green vegetables.

Inositol

Inositol works with choline to keep the bloodstream in a healthy condition. It's one of the "youth" vitamins, along with pantothenic acid and PABA, since it slows down hardening of the arteries. Too much coffee or tea can keep the inositol in the diet from being absorbed because the caffeine reacts with it. In males, lecithin is an important part of the sexual fluid so a combination of lecithin and phosphatidyl choline is a vital step in keeping their sexual level at a peak.

Food sources are sesame seeds, whole grains, blackstrap molasses, eggs, legumes, grapefruit.

Vitamin B^{12}

This vitamin is the only one that is a combination of vitamin and mineral. It has a molecule of cobalt at its center. It is needed for the manufacture of nucleic acid (DNA) and the myelin sheath that covers and protects the nerves. Lecithin and cholesterol also contribute to the protective effort. B^{12} is essential to the metabolism of proteins, fats and carbohydrates. Every cell in the body needs vitamin B^{12}.

A B^{12}-deficiency-induced anemia will cut down the sex drive enormously and the nerve problems created by a deficiency will also create great sexual difficulties. If there is a deficiency of iron, B^6 and/or calcium, B^{12} will not be easily absorbed from food.

Early symptoms include fatigue, irritability, slow thinking ability, menstrual disturbances, paleness, muscle jerking and mental problems that can range from mild symptoms to severe ones. Even in the early stages, a B^{12} deficiency can play havoc with your sex life so insure a good supply either from the diet or with a supplement.

Good food sources include lean meats, liver, fish, poultry, eggs, cheese, milk, yogurt, seaweed and a one-celled organism known as chlorella (available in health food stores in tablet form).

This ends the coverage of the B-complex vitamins. Most vitamin formulas will deliver all of the B-vitamins in one tablet or capsule. Many stores carry either a B-complex 50 or B-complex 100. This will give you 100 (or 50) milligrams of the B-vitamins. In the case of biotin, B^{12} and folic acid, the dosage will be in micrograms. Some companies offer a different delivery system, a time-release B-complex, which is the better formula since it releases the vitamins over an 8 to 10 hour span of time.

Vitamin C

This vitamin is very important to the body for many reasons, but we'll concentrate on how it affects your sex life. It is water soluble, like the B-complex vitamins, and is easily lost in cooking, so you have to supply the body with all it needs every day. There's a lot of differing opinion about the amount needed. Some experts say you should have 2 to 3 grams (2,000 to 3,000 milligrams) a day. Some say up to 10 grams daily (Dr. Linus Pauling), while others say you need only 50 mg to 100 mg.

(My personal preference is for 2,000 to 3,000 milligrams in a time-release form.)

Vitamin C promotes better use of vitamins A, B-complex, E, iron and calcium. This can have a direct effect on your sex life because its role in iron utilization and the formation of blood cells is directly connected with energy. It is a necessary vitamin for the adrenal glands. The adrenals make hormones and neurotransmitters which exert profound influence on sexual activity. One of the adrenal hormones is involved in precipitating an orgasm.

Vitamin C also contributes to good sex by helping to keep our bodies limber and active, and by helping to keep arteries clear as it works against cholesterol buildup.

The body usually has about 5 grams of vitamin C circulating around. Some comes from food and the rest from supplements. But, if you smoke, are stressed, have a fever, take aspirin, or take antibiotics, you cut down on the vitamin C that is available.

Good food sources are citrus fruits, tomatoes, mangoes, strawberries, avocados and Brussels sprouts.

Vitamin D

Called the "sunshine vitamin" because, when the sun's rays strike capillaries near the skin's surface, a certain type of cholesterol in the blood is converted into vitamin D. But, this is not the best way to get vitamin D in our modern times. In much older times the human race spent a lot of time in the sun without clothing, and there was little smoke or smog to interfere with the body's manufacture of vitamin D. If you think how little time we spend in the sun, unclothed, during the year, it makes sense to take supplements that supply vitamin D. Cod liver oil is one of the best, since you will get vitamins A and D together.

Vitamin D controls blood calcium and the ratio of calcium to phosphorus. Choline and lecithin contain phosphorus which is needed for sex play. If the ratio is disturbed by a deficiency of vitamin D, more phosphorus may be excreted which would call for a breakdown of lecithin and choline. This would work against your sexual desire and enjoyment.

Vitamin D is found in liver, fish, butter and eggs. Although Cod Liver Oil is a good source of vitamin D and comes in tablet and capsule form as well as liquid, it is not the same as the fish oil which is the supplemental source of EPA and DSA (the fish oil supplement usually called MAX EPA). A good routine is to take Cod Liver Oil three times a week with meals for vitamin D and to take MAX EPA (two capsules with each meal) every day.

More mature individuals, especially during the winter months, should be sure to get plenty of vitamin D since calcium intake, vitamin D and strong bones go together. Women, in particular, take note of the calcium/vitamin D connection.

Vitamin E

This vitamin does a great job in protecting fatty acids from being over-burned (oxidation). Since fatty acids play a part in the production of sex hormones, if there isn't enough vitamin E running around in your body, then there won't be enough sex hormones doing the same.

Vitamins A and C are also protected by vitamin E and, since both of them are involved in satisfying sex, this is another reason to have enough E in the body.

Vitamin E was first named by the Greeks who called it *tocopherols,* which means "to assist childbirth," because they discovered that it was necessary to the reproductive system of animals.

Its protective action extends to hormones from the pituitary and adrenal glands and to the heart muscle. It helps the cells of your muscles breathe, and therefore increases their energy.

Most experts agree that the natural form of vitamin E has more activity than the synthetic form so ask before you buy.

Food sources can include eggs, cheese, liver, leeks, cabbage, Brussels sprouts, wheat germ, raw nuts and seeds, parsley, dill and dandelion, but it's hard to insure a good supply unless you take supplemental vitamin E.

Most vitamin/mineral formulas contain vitamin E in its natural state, at least those you buy in the health food stores. Some companies use the synthetic form because it is cheaper. The synthetic vitamin E will do the job but you need more of it than you do of the natural E.

Remember, you can't spell SEX without the E!

Vitamin F

There is no such vitamin as vitamin F but nutritionists call it that instead of essential fatty acids because it's easier to say.

Essential fatty acids are found in vegetable oils. They are linoleic acid, linolenic acid and arachidonic acid. We can't manufacture these acids but must obtain them from foods.

Vitamin F is necessary for the manufacture of prostaglandins (the hormone-like substances which govern so much activity in the body), and is needed by the thyroid gland, the adrenal glands and the prostate gland. It promotes calcium absorption, helps to slow down cholesterol buildup, helps regulate blood coagulation and aids in membrane making.

It also is important to beauty as well as health since it helps to keep hair lustrous and skin moist. Many hair and skin problems can be corrected by using a tablespoonful of vegetable oil and apple cider vinegar on a fresh green salad daily.

If you do that and also take two fish oil capsules with meals you will insure a steady supply of the raw material your body must have to stay healthy and sexy.

Vitamin K

This vitamin is included just to keep the record straight. It is necessary to keep your clotting mechanism in good order but has little to do with your sex life. As long as you establish an eating habit which includes cabbage, spinach, cauliflower, you'll stay in good vitamin K shape.

Vitamins Get the Headlines But Minerals Are Just as Important

According to the Bible, man was made from clay. Clay is basically composed of minerals but we can't eat clay and take the minerals into our system. We have to depend on plants to take in the minerals from the clay and convert them into edible and absorbable compounds. You can't eat iron directly from an iron mine but you can eat spinach which contains iron and get the nutrient metal that way.

If we don't eat enough vegetables we have to take mineral supplements. These supplements supply minerals in a form that is the same as that supplied by nature or as close as possible. Iron, for example, is best taken as an organic compound (ferrous gluconate) or as a chelate (surrounded by organic material such as an amino acid). Inorganic iron, such as ferrous sulfate, is much harsher to the stomach — frequently causing upset — and is more difficult to absorb.

Most mineral formulas take into consideration the best type of combination and try to present all of the minerals in their most absorbable form.

This section will examine minerals as they affect your sex life, leaving a lot of their action in the body for further reading by yourself. There are many books devoted to vitamin and mineral activity and you should read as much as you can about how they help you on an overall basis.

Calcium

There has been a spate of publicity about this mineral because of its relation to osteoporosis and strong bones. It is the most abundant mineral in the body. It is also one of the most deficient in the diets of Americans. Calcium is needed for building bones, teeth, and other body cells. It helps maintain the acid-alkaline balance in the blood and is so important that the body will "rob" calcium from bones if it is needed in other places in the body.

Calcium affects the production of hormones from the endocrine glands. This, in turn, helps control the menstrual cycle and fertility. It is necessary for lactation, the healthy functioning of muscles (including the heart muscle) and nerves. Calcium contributes forcefully to stamina and energy, particularly important to love play. It also contributes to the relaxation that follows a successful sexual encounter.

Glandular instability due to a deficiency of calcium will lead to a loss of sexual ability and a loss of sexual interest.

Prior to menopause, calcium is needed to help prevent PMS. After menopause, it is needed to prevent bone loss and osteoporosis. A combination of calcium obtained from the diet and from supplements should equal at least 1,000 milligrams a day. That amount should rise to 1,250 milligrams daily after menopause.

For the best benefits, calcium should be taken in supplement form, along with vitamin D, magnesium, vitamin C, and boron (3 mg) to insure its assimilation.

Calcium-containing foods include milk products, raw nuts and seeds, whole grains, green leafy vegetables, onions, fish, meat, eggs, brown rice and seaweed.

Even if you think you eat a diet which provides most of the calcium needed for your continued good health and good sex, it's a good idea to use a supplement once or twice a day for insurance.

Silica

Silica is found in abundance in the clay of the earth and we need silica for good health. It helps bones to knit, makes your skin, nails and hair glow with health and be sensitive to the touch of love. Silica also helps make the sheaths that cover the nerves.

Although you can obtain silica from lettuce, whole grains, sprouts and brown rice, it's a good idea to use a supplement daily. Vegetable silica from the herb Equisetum is available in 8 grain capsules (520 milligrams) at most health food stores.

Sodium

We hear about sodium in the negative most of the time because a lot of Americans salt their food too much, or eat foods that have previously been salted too much by the manufacturer. This excess salt holds water in the body and contributes to high blood pressure.

Excess salt is no good for you but some sodium is necessary to equalize acids in the body and help keep joints and ligaments flexible. It is also involved in nerve conduction.

All of your sexual fluids involve sodium salts.

Salt is sodium chloride, but is a poor source of this important mineral. It's found in many foods so you don't really have to supplement to get enough. Just eat a healthful diet of greens, raw nuts and seeds, some fish and some seaweed.

Potassium

Your heart muscle and skeletal muscles need potassium in order to respond to the body's directives. If you lack a sufficient supply, your sexual control is apt to go haywire. Weakness and a lack of coordination would make you sexually awkward. Vitality, strength, rhythmic movement all depend on potassium.

Foods which contain potassium in large supply are bananas, raw nuts and seeds, wheat bran, wheat germ, blackstrap molasses, lima beans and parsley.

If you take a diuretic drug (water pill), your doctor will advise a potassium supplement but usually your food will supply all that you need.

A good multivitamin/mineral supplement will include a supply of potassium balanced to the intake of the other minerals present.

Ask at your health food store counter or read the label carefully.

Iron

Women need iron. Particularly before the menopause. Iron is part of the red blood cell and it carries life-giving oxygen throughout the body.

Without enough iron present you will be fatigued and lose all interest in sex. Iron is vital to an enjoyable sex life.

The fact that iron is difficult to absorb and assimilate contributes to a possible deficiency. If you take an iron supplement, see that it also contains some vitamin C or drink orange juice when you take it.

Eat liver, eggs, green leafy vegetables, asparagus, almonds, fish, poultry, prunes, raisins, apricots, cherries and raspberries. It's hard to get enough iron in your life so watch out for a lack of this mineral.

Phosphorus

No phosphorus . . . no sex!

That's the bottom line.

Phosphorus is essential to your brain and nerve activity, and the two of them are essential to sex.

Fortunately for the human race, there is seldom a shortage of this essential mineral. It's found in eggs, seafood, meat, poultry, seeds and nuts, whole grains, brown rice, legumes, cabbage and corn.

Lecithin is loaded with phosphorus. Take two capsules of lecithin, 1200 milligrams each, with each meal. It will increase sexual arousal and then build more enjoyment into every act. Take phosphatidyl choline (Phos-Chol) once or twice a day for additional support because phosphorus is also one of the main constituents of bones and teeth.

You can get your supplements at health food stores or at some drugstores.

Sulfur

Sulfur is one of the elements that keeps brains and nerves working at top capacity. Some of the other minerals that share the burden are manganese, silica and phosphorus.

Sulfur also helps to keep skin and hair younger looking. It is a cleansing agent and keeps your sex organs free of impurities so they can perform at a higher level.

Sulfur and molasses used to be a common spring event in the late 1800's and early 1900's but its bad taste have made it only a memory for today's people. Eat eggs, garlic, onions, leeks, cauliflower, broccoli, Brussels sprouts, asparagus, cabbage, kale, radishes, and turnips instead.

Iodine

This mineral is chiefly used by the thyroid gland which is the gland controlling metabolism. Iodine is instrumental in regulating the production and utilization of energy. You wouldn't be able to think, speak, act, without this mineral being present in abundant amounts.

The growth of your hair, skin, teeth and nails is iodine-dependent. All of this is due to the place played by iodine in the production of the very important hormone called thyroxine.

A deficiency can cause irritability, depression, malaise, lack of energy, and even bone disturbances since iodine is also involved in calcium metabolism.

Stress depletes the body's iodine supplies resulting in a loss of sex drive and menstrual problems.

Eat seafood, kelp, dulse, pineapple, or get some kelp tablets at your health food store if you find that you are suffering from an iodine deficiency.

It is difficult for you to tell if you are suffering from an iodine deficiency or any other mineral deficiency. It may be necessary for you to consult with a health professional and take various tests. However, if you find you have some of the symptoms and decide to try doing the test yourself by buying some kelp tablets and trying them for six weeks to see the results, it might be the easiest way to restore your sex drive and your zest for life.

Check the label and follow the directions.

Manganese

Manganese takes part in a number of enzyme reactions and is very important to the nerves and the brain's operation. It is essential in human sexuality. If manganese is lacking in the diet, there will be little interest in the mating game.

Foods containing manganese are whole grains, green vegetables, eggs, nuts and seeds, pineapple and apricots.

Most good multiple vitamin/mineral formulas contain some manganese to help make up for shortages in the diet.

Magnesium

Magnesium has the power to relax you and relaxation is the key to better sex. You can't expect good sexual relations if you are stressed, tense, angry, etc. Magnesium, in good supply, enhances your ability to initiate and enjoy sexual contact.

It is found in leafy green vegetables, nuts and seeds, wheat germ, whole grains, seafood, kelp, legumes, milk and meat.

It is always found in multiple vitamin/mineral formulas. The best amount is usually half as much as the amount of calcium in the formula.

Chromium

Usually found in formulas as GTF chromium, it helps the body utilize insulin and regulates blood sugar. (More about this element later on in this part.)

Food sources include seafood, meat, milk products, Brewer's yeast, seaweeds.

Since there is a chance of a deficiency, supplementation is the best insurance.

Selenium

Works alongside vitamin E to promote fertility and to protect the unsaturated fatty acids from oxidation. It contributes to healthy, young looking skin.

Food sources include cereals, grains, fish, broccoli, onions, garlic and tomatoes.

Zinc

Zinc has hundreds of jobs in the body, including the proper maintenance of the sexual system. A loss of zinc is related to a loss of the sex drive and zinc is one of the most important of the minerals related to good sex.

Zinc-containing foods include oysters, eggs, nuts and seeds and whole grains. However, supplementation is advised for insurance.

The following pages contain listings of all the major vitamins and minerals, their sources and their functions.

Vitamin Sources and Functions

Vitamin	Source	Function
Vitamin A (Retinol)	Fish, fish-liver oils, liver, meat, eggs, cheese, yogurt.	Sex hormone production; protection of nasal, respiratory and vaginal membranes.
Pro-Vitamin A (Carotene)	Leafy green vegetables, yellow fruits and vegetables, broccoli, peas.	Converted to vitamin A.
Vitamin B^1 (Thiamine)	Raw nuts and seeds, asparagus, beans, pineapple, soybeans, yogurt, wheat germ, whole grains, herbs, liver, meat, fish roe.	Energy production, aids overall metabolism.
Vitamin B^2 (Riboflavin)	Milk, organ meats, baby green vegetables, raw nuts and seeds, wheat germ, rice polishings, broccoli, asparagus,soybeans,herbs.	Energy production, healing of wounds.
Vitamin B^3 (Niacin)	Meat, chicken, fish, asparagus, dates, raw almonds, bran, wheat germ, rice polishings, broccoli, yogurt, raw seeds, herbs.	Aids circulatory and digestive system function.
Vitamin B^6 (Pyridoxine)	Wheat germ, wheat bran, rice polishings, whole grains, organ meats, raw nuts and seeds, eggs, honey, molasses.	Aids metabolism of amino acids; aids in brain function.

Vitamin	Source	Function
Pantothenic Acid (B vitamin Category)	Organ meats, milk, eggs, whole grains, raw nuts and seeds, poultry, fish, molasses, broccoli, cabbage, cauliflower.	Aids in production of red blood cells, steroid hormones, and overall energy.
Biotin (B vitamin category)	Cereals, vegetables, milk, liver, raw egg whites.	May alleviate symptoms of depression.
PABA (B vitamin Category)	See Folic Acid.	Involved in production of folic acid; aids function of bowels, hair, skin; nearly always found with folic acid.
Folic Acid (B vitamin Category)	Liver, leafy green vegetables, broccoli, Brussels sprouts, raw nuts and seeds, asparagus, sprouts.	Involved in maintenance of chromosomes; safeguards against anemia.
Choline (B vitamin Category)	Egg yolk, meat, poultry, fish, fish roe, soybeans, whole grains, green vegetables.	Aids in production of neurotransmitters; aids in function of circulatory system and kidney function.
Inositol (B vitamin Category)	Sesame seed butter, tahini, beef heart, whole grains, blackstrap molasses, soybeans, grapefruit, legumes, eggs, fish roe.	See Choline.

Vitamin	Source	Function
Vitamin B^{12}	Meat, organ meats, fish, poultry, eggs, cheese, milk, yogurt, chlorella, seaweed.	Aids in DNA synthesis; metabolizes proteins, carbohyrates, fats; prevents anemia.
Vitamin C	Acerola, strawberries, tomatoes, mangoes, avocados, Brussels sprouts.	Promotes absorption of other vitamins, iron, calcium; necessary for function of adrenal glands; protects body against stress.
Vitamin D	Fish, butter, eggs, liver, fish-liver oils.	Controls calcium levels.
Vitamin E	Eggs, fish roe, cheese, sardines, liver, soybeans, leeks, cabbage, Brussels sprouts, herbs, raw wheat germ; nuts, seeds, and sprouts.	Protects fatty acids from oxidizing; aids in sex hormone production; reduces ugly vein congestion.
Vitamin F	Raw seeds and nuts, whole grains, wheat germ, whole milk, vegetable oils.	Aids in function of thyroid, adrenal, and prostate gland; manufactures prostaglandins; promotes calcium absorption; slows cholesterol build-up
Vitamin K	Kidneys, cabbage, soybeans, spinach, cauliflower.	Aids in formation of Prothrombin, a blood-clotting factor.

Mineral Sources and Functions

Mineral	Source	Function
Calcium	Whole raw milk, yogurt, cheese, raw nuts and seeds, whole grains, green vegetables (especially kale).	Maintains acid/alkaline balance; aids function of heart, muscles, and nerves; helps form bone.
Silicon	Oat straw tea, sprouts, rice polishings, whole grains.	Protects and strengthens nerves, hair, skin, nails.
Sodium	Veal joint broth, goat milk, okra, celery.	Aids function of digestive and lymphatic systems; component of blood; maintains nerve conduction and electromagnetic potential of tissues.
Potassium	Blackstrap molasses, soybeans, dried fruits, bananas, raw seeds and nuts, lima beans, rice and wheat bran, wheat germ, parsley, lentils, spinach, avocados, meat.	Electrochemical balance of tissues of heart and muscles.
Iron	Organ meats, egg yolks, green leafy vegetables, almonds, fish, asparagus, poultry, bing cherries, black raspberries, prunes, raisins, apricots.	Component of red blood cells; transports oxygen to lungs; aids in cell respiration.
Phosphorus	Brain: Egg yolks, codfish roe, seafood, raw milk. Bones: Vegetables, seeds and nuts, whole grains, rice polishings, wheat bran, legumes, cabbage, corn.	Essential to brain and nerve function.

Mineral	Source	Function
Oxygen	Air, small amounts of solid and liquid food.	Not a mineral. Most important element of life.
Sulfur	Egg yolk, onion, garlic, leeks, cauliflower, broccoli, Brussels sprouts, asparagus, cabbage, kale, figs, parsnips, radishes, spinach, turnips.	Aids function of brain and nerves; a body cleanser.
Iodine	Seafood, dulse, kelp, pineapple, foods grown near the ocean.	Fuels thyroid gland, which controls the body's metabolism.
Magnesium	Leafy green vegetables, yellow cornmeal, raw nuts and seeds, wheat germ, whole grains, seafood, kelp, dulse, legumes, milk, meat.	Aids in muscle relaxation, protein synthesis, energy production; natural laxative.
Manganese	Whole grains, green vegetables, egg yolk, raw nuts and seeds, Missouri black walnuts, pineapple, apples, apricots.	Necessary in enzyme, brain function.
Chromium (Micronutrient)	Seafood, meat, whole grains, corn oil.	Aids in regulation of blood sugar levels.
Cobalt (Micronutrient)	Seafood, meat, milk products, Sun, chlorella, seaweed.	Aids in formation of red blood cells, function of enzymes and nerves.
Copper (Micronutrient)	Organ meats, green vegetables, raw nuts and seeds, whole grains.	Aids in formation of red blood cells and hemoglobin.

Mineral	Source	Function
Germanium (Micronutrient)	Garlic, ginseng, aloe vera, comfrey, green leafy vegetables.	Aids in function of immune system and bowels; may help alleviate mood disorders.
Selenium (Micronutrient)	Cereal brans and germs, broccoli, onions, ocean fish, tomatoes.	Works with vitamin E to delay oxidation of fatty acids and promotes fertility.
Zinc	Organ meats, oysters, fish roe, whole grain cereals, raw nuts and seeds (especially pumpkin seeds).	Maintains health levels of sexual system in both males and females.

12

FOOD, SUPPLEMENTS, PLANTS, HERBS AND ESSENTIAL OILS TO FUEL YOUR SEX MACHINE

Good sex needs fuel and you can get it from a combination of food and supplements. If your calories are too low because you're on too stringent a fasting diet, you won't have the energy for a good "roll in the hay." But, a reduced-calorie diet that increases your sexual vigor makes you slim and trim and lets you have fun in the sun and in the bedroom!

What Are The Staple Sexy Foods?

Beans, vegetables, fish, nuts and seeds. They're rich in vitamin E (needed for the production of the sex hormones), zinc (for the hormonal balance), trace elements and all of the B-vitamins just described.

A strong multi-vitamin/mineral will add insurance, but here's seven days of sexy foods to start you off.

A Seven Day Diet of Sexy Foods

Monday

Breakfast

Peel an orange for breakfast

Then eat a whole-grain cereal with raisins, nuts, dried fruit and skim milk, with cinnamon dusted on top

Finish with a slice of whole wheat bread lightly toasted and a glass of water

Lunch

Peanut butter on 1 slice of "Brannola" or whole wheat bread

A green salad

Some fruit sherbert (any flavor)

1 cup of skim milk

Dinner

1/2 dozen raw oysters soaking in lemon juice

1/2 cup potato salad and 1 cup raw broccoli (make a dressing of olive oil and apple cider vinegar), follow with herbal tea

Tuesday

Breakfast

Melon balls

1 slice of rye bread with 1 ounce of cheddar cheese

1 cup of skim milk

Lunch

Get a whole wheat pita and fill it with sprouts and tuna fish

Eat an apple

Drink 1 cup of skim milk

Dinner

Fresh Gazpacho soup

Make a salad of mushrooms, 1 hard-boiled egg, 2 bacon slices (drained), 1 cup of fresh, raw spinach and a cup of snap beans

Herbal tea

Snack on a cup of plain yogurt

Wednesday

Breakfast

Orange juice for a starter

Slap some farmer cheese on cinnamon toast

Have a cup of coffee for a change with 1/2 skim milk

Lunch

Whole wheat pita loaded with onion and sprouts plus a slice of tofu

Green salad — your choice of fresh greens with apple cider vinegar and olive oil dressing

Mix plain yogurt and some fresh strawberries

Dinner

1/2 dozen raw oysters soaking in lemon juice

1/2 cup potato salad and 1 cup raw broccoli (make a dressing of olive oil and apple cider vinegar), follow with herbal tea

Thursday

Breakfast

Any whole wheat cereal with fruit topping

Cup of skim milk

Lunch

Salmon salad with onions, celery, peppers

1 slice of rye bread

1 whole peach (fresh)

1 cup of skim milk

Dinner

6 ounces of shrimp any way you like them

Peas, tomato and onion salad

2 slices of whole wheat bread

Herbal tea

Snack on some yogurt

Friday

Breakfast

Try grapefruit for a change. Either 1/2 a grapefruit or a glass of juice

Cheddar cheese on whole wheat toast

1 cup of skim milk

Lunch

Vegetable salad (raw) with a couple of hard-boiled eggs

1 slice of bread (rye, pumpernickel or whole wheat)

Fruit salad

1 cup of skim milk

Dinner

Treat yourself to steamed mussels
Lettuce, carrot and chick pea salad
1 slice bread
1/2 cup yogurt with some fresh fruit topping
Herbal tea

Snack on a pear

Saturday

Breakfast

Mix some fruit or some grapefruit and orange sections
Scrambled eggs with chopped onions
1 corn muffin
1 cup skim milk

Lunch

Yogurt and banana mixture
A couple of crackers (no salt)
Herbal tea

Dinner

Lemon sole with onions and garlic
4 ounces of wild rice
Zucchini salad (raw) with sweet onions
Herbal tea

Sunday

Breakfast

Buckwheat pancakes with a drop of maple syrup
Juice
1 cup of skim milk

Lunch

Chicken (no skin)
Sprout and fresh vegetable salad
Whole wheat bread
1 cup of skim milk

Dinner

4 ounce hamburger
Brussels sprouts with mustard sauce
Green salad
Herbal tea

Snack on an apple

(Feed your partner the same diet. This is for both males and females. No sense your feeling "in the mood" if he's dragging his behind.)

Plant Essence Therapy

Herbal therapy has been one of the healing methods since the dawn of time but the use of healing essences from flowers and herbs, drawn from them during a distilling process, is a much newer therapy.

The parts of the plant which contain most of the odorous material that gives the plant its particular odor (the petals of the rose, the bark of the sandalwood tree or the rind of the lemon) is distilled and the volatile oil is captured. It is a lot like a perfume but much more concentrated. It should always be diluted if it is to be used on the skin and only tiny amounts are ever used.

These plant essences can alleviate minor health problems, improve the appearance of your skin and hair and definitely enhance your sensuality.

Few people know the magic of plant essence. This next section will introduce you to some of the magical properties and how you can use them to your advantage for healing and for more pleasurable experiences.

Too Tired for a Matinee?

Experts tell us that one of the best times for lovemaking is in the morning but what if you constantly wake up feeling irritable and lethargic?

Try something new!

Run a medium hot bath, add two drops of rosemary and two drops of clary sage. Stir the water. Get in and soak for fifteen minutes. Inhale the heady scent.

Then, get out . . . dry yourself and slip back in bed with whomever.

The same clary sage can be of great help during an emotional trauma attack. A drop or two on a tissue can turn an "off" day into an "on" day. In fact, because it is an essential oil known as a euphoric oil, it can make you quite "high."

Muscles too Tired to be Sexually Responsive?

Have him give you a sensual rubdown as part of foreplay. It's something different and may stimulate an old marriage into a new delight.

Mix the following in advance and keep it near your bed—

Juniper oil	10 drops
Lavender oil	6 drops
Rosemary oil	8 drops

Vegetable oil, enough to bring the total amount to two ounces

Have him rub your legs, arms and back. You'll know when the aches have gone and you're ready for love.

Do Your Feet Hurt?

Get a bowl and fill it with warm water. Add six drops of peppermint oil. Put your aching feet into the mixture and either you or a companion can gently massage them. A few minutes of massage should help, and don't forget to include the soles of your feet. The reflex zones on the soles connect to many sensuous areas which respond to gentle rubbing.

Too Tense for Sex?

When you're tight as a drum, sex is the last thing on your mind. Unwind in minutes with the therapy of a warm bath treated with an essential oil. Many people reach for the prescription bottle and a tranquilizer but being tranquilized doesn't make sex better. The soaking in a scented bath is mentally and physically therapeutic, and if you share the bath with your old or new lover, so much the better.

Try a few drops of germanium or neroli or lavender and feel the tension evaporate into the water, to be flushed down the drain as you begin to flush with other thoughts. For those extra special nights use oil of ylang-ylang.

No side effects and non-addictive, and your senses are heightened not deadened.

PMS? Take a Bath

That's right. If PMS makes you tense and irritable, upset and teary, take a bath. Use a drop or two of lavender or clary sage in the warm water and take a twenty minute relaxing dunk. Keep a drop of clary sage on a tissue through the day. It'll help you to keep a lot of troubles away.

What You Put On Can Make or Break A Sexual Encounter

Not clothes but scents.

Many essences excite the senses. The sense of smell is vital to sexual awareness. We can close our eyes and turn off the room in favor of our imagination, but we can't turn off our noses. Put some ylang-ylang, jasmine, patchouli or sandalwood on a light bulb or sprinkle some around the room. Or put a drop on yourself in some strategic spots. Vary your scent to give a different illusion. Variety can be a turn on.

Can Essential Oils Help Enlarge Your Breasts?

Plant hormones (called phytosterols) may work in ways similar to human hormones which help develop the breasts. The blend of oils that follows is gently massaged in for a few minutes morning and night and can have a pleasing effect. That's all there is to it. And it's even better if you have someone to help with the massage.

Try this mixture:

Germanium	8 drops
Ylang-Ylang	14 drops

Vegetable oil, enough to bring the mixture up to 2 ounces

The Rub-Away-Fat Formula

You will lose weight when you diet and a slim, hard body is more conducive to romance than a fat, flabby one, but diet alone will not reduce those fat thighs and rear end. Exercise is a must for tonifying and firming up. However, the regular use of an essential oil formula will help to remove superfluous fat from regions that don't get too much exercise even when you exercise. Stroke the area in an upwards direction from knees to hips for one week out of a month.

Don't pinch, pummel or treat the skin in a rough manner. Just a gentle, upwards massage.

Use the following mixture:

Juniper 10 drops

Cypress 10 drops

Vegetable oil, enough to bring the mixture up to 2 ounces

Good Scents Make for Good Sex and Vice Versa

Back in the cave days, before we knew that sex was for fun as well as to make babies, there had to be some method for the cave man to know when the best time for procreation had arrived. So nature arranged for odors and gave the orgasm as a reward for following her orders.

Just in case you think all this is made up, science is beginning to investigate the way scents affect people by using the Electroencephalograph (EEG). Yale psychophysiologist Gary Schwartz studied the effect of spiced-apple fragrance on volunteers hooked up to the EEG. He found that blood pressure and heart rates were lowered and their breathing slowed which indicated to him that the scent had generated relaxation. This is only the first case of investigation into the way scents can affect the brain, but it is not the last.

Susan Schiffman, a professor of medical psychology at Duke Medical Center explains that the early cortex (part of the brain) that we inherited from our ancestors, which has to do with the sense of smell, also has to do with the limbic region of the brain, the emotional center. So when you smell something, it generally triggers an emotional memory.

Soviet scientists, experimenting with scents such as mint, lavender, sage and anis, said they improved the alertness and work capacity of air traffic controllers. The controllers said they felt fresher and were able to work longer without fatigue.

Scents have been incorporated into many healing modalities. For example: eucalyptus oil is used in chest rubs because the odor helps bring up phlegm. Oils of anise, clove, peppermint and chamomile have been used in toothpaste because they are antiseptic in nature. Birch oil and oils of thyme and oregano are often used in limiments because of their abilities to soothe muscular aches. Clove oil has been used in dentistry for centuries.

RESOURCES

Alexandra Avery Purely
Natural Body Care
Northrup Creek
Clatskanie, OR 970160
(503) 755-2446

Aphrodisia
282 Bleeker St.
New York, NY 10014
(212) 989-6400

Aroma Vera, Inc.
P.O. Box 3609
Culver City, CA 90231
(213) 973-4253

Attar
Playground Rd.
New Ipswich, NH 03701
(603) 878-1780

Bonne Sante Health Products
462 62nd St.
Brooklyn, NY 11220
(718) 492-3887

The Chishti Company
P.O. Box 79
New Virginia Road
Oxford, NY 13830
(800) 344-7172
(607) 843-9644

Ledet Oils
P.O. Box 2354
Fair Oaks, CA 95628
(916) 965-7546

Original Swiss Aromatics
P.O. Box 606
San Rafael, CA 94915
(415) 459-3998

Aura Cacia
P.O. Box 391
Weaverville, CA 96093
(707) 584-5115

Talisman
68 Tinker St.
Woodstock, NY 10003
(914) 679-7647

If your local store does not stock these oils, you can write for a catalog to buy them through the mail, or by phone.

13

PMS

A Very Real and Very Regular Form of Suffering

It is a major cause of social problems.

It is a major cause of divorce, marital strife, juvenile delinquency.

It will utterly destroy a sexual relationship because you don't want to have sex when troubled with PMS, and your lover or husband, because of abuse, wants nothing to do with you when you're feeling better!

Estrogen has been promoted as a therapy for PMS on the most dubious of grounds. But estrogen can cause more problems than it corrects.

It can cause a magnesium deficiency which promotes clotting (*Amer. J. Clin. Nutr.* 27, pp. 59-79, 1974). The magnesium deficiency can also promote abnormal fat metabolism.

Estrogens are not useful if taken over a long period of time but natural supplements can be of fantastic help.

The following pages will tell you how to recognize PMS when you have it.

How to minimize its effects with vitamins, amino acids and other nutrients.

How to use a special anti-PMS diet.

How to minimize contributory stress.

After reading and using the advice for a period of only 90 days, you may be able to enjoy sex right up to the last second of your life.

It Took Two Murders

Suddenly the world began talking about a disease that didn't exist in the eyes of most medical practitioners. A stunned public was forced to consider the facts when informed that a British court had reduced two murder charges to manslaughter because the accused murderers, two women, had been shown to have had "diminished responsibility" due to PMS.

Why did it take so long and have to cause two deaths before a syndrome as old as man- and womankind could be publicized?

Why, almost fifty years after PMS was meticulously explained by Dr. Robert T. Frank of New York in a now-famous thesis, "The Hormonal Causes of Premenstrual Tension," is this syndrome being exploited as though it just appeared on the scene? A half century ago, Dr. Frank had observed premenstrual disturbances that ranged from minor problems of fatigue and lack of concentration to major concerns such as epileptic-like convulsions, asthma, and depression severe enough to make the sufferer contemplate taking her own life. It should have been a medical breakthrough, but it hardly caused a ripple in an ocean of unconcern.

Consider the following from gynecological textbooks published between 1952 and 1978:

Novak and Novak, *Textbook of Gynecology:*

> While many women suffer no discomfort whatsoever during menstruation, a moderate amount of pelvic heaviness and even an occasional cramp may be considered as within normal limits.
>
> It needs no more than a knowledge of human nature to justify the statement that the same degree of peripheral stimulation which, in the well balanced, phlegmatic individual will be expressed as a moderate discomfort, *will manifest itself in the high-strung supersensitive girl by severe and incapacitating pain.*
>
> The psychogenic element . . . may accentuate the subjective element in a particular case. Among these are a *congenitally unstable and high strung nervous system, psychic trauma, especially when related to the menstrual period, and*

wrong ideas as to the significance and normality of the menstrual function.

Brewer, *Textbook of Gynecology:*

Psychogenic causes are the most common and the most important in cases of primary dysmenorrhea.

It is common that a mother, *who herself is not adjusted,* transmits to her daughter the feeling that menstruation is a period of being unwell. *Menstruation also lends itself as an excuse for avoiding things that are undesired.*

In most girls, menstruation is associated with great anxiety, fear and uncertainty. *If an individual happens to be unstable emotionally,* these are all enhanced. *Most reactions could be obviated by proper counseling prior to puberty.* This would reduce the frequency of dysmenorrhea to a large extent. The threshold for pain varies greatly. Most women have some local pelvic sensation at the time of menstruation. *To some this is interpreted as pain, whereas others are capable of ignoring it completely.*

(Emphasis added by the author in all cases.)

In general, most textbook references to menstrual pain are pretty much the same. Women are labeled hysterical and traditionally they have accepted the diagnosis, along with the pain and discomfort. But in most instances, it is *men* who wrote the textbooks and trained the physicians, and it is as difficult for them to accept new ideas about PMS as it is to accept nutritional treatments for it.

But beware: the impetus for the sudden interest in PMS may not be entirely due to concern with the relief of symptoms. Lawyers brought PMS into the public awareness because it was connected to murder, and the press corps, mostly male, may be anxious to expose a uniquely female condition that might imply that women are unfit to be decision makers. The purpose here is therefore to describe the different facets of Premenstrual Syndrome and suggest possible nutritional alternatives to traditional drug therapy. Politics are best left to the politicians.

"The Curse"

Way back in time, it was easy to consider menstruation as a magical event. The cave man could only consider loss of blood to be connected with loss of life, and to watch a woman bleed for five or six days every month without dying must have been awesome and even frightening.

Civilization progressed but menstrual facts remained in the caves. The word "menstruation" is derived from the Latin "mens" meaning month. But month was derived from moon and in Greek, "moon" is "mene." To the ancients, menses were cosmically controlled like the phases of the moon. It was logical, therefore, to assume that anything connected with menstruation was also controlled by the cosmos.

Many ancient religions, and some of those practiced today, viewed and still view this natural, healthy occurrence as repugnant. Moslem women are not allowed to enter the holy mosques when menstruating. In the Orthodox Jewish faith, a woman's "clean" days are after her period and after a purifying bath. The early Catholic church forbade sexual congress during menses, calling it a sin, while the Greek Orthodox faith would not offer a woman communion during her menstrual period.

Superstition kept menstruating women away from the barn for fear they would curdle the milk, and French and German women were forbidden to enter wineries because they might sour the wine or beer. In *The Second Sex,* Simone de Beauvoir says that in France it is widely believed that menstruating women have a bad effect on cider fermentation, the curing of bacon and the refining of sugar.

Myths, superstitions and ignorance in many countries have perpetuated the notion that the wondrous internal cleansing activity is a "curse," and have brainwashed women into accepting a falsehood as reality.

Physical and Mental Symptoms

In 1931, Dr. Frank read what should have been a history-making paper at a meeting of the Section of Neurology and Psychiatry at the New York Academy of Medicine. Shortly after it was presented, it was published in *Archives of Neurology and Psychiatry.* Although

Dr. Frank brilliantly focused on a medical condition that needed scientific recognition, it remained for another doctor, Guy E. Abraham, M.D., a former professor of obstetrics, gynecology and endocrinology at UCLA, to associate PMS with a group of symptoms and to advise nutritional support to relieve each group.

Dr. Abraham feels that PMS must be considered a disease and treated as such. According to him, "It is a very real and very regular form of suffering for some nine to twelve million women. In my opinion, PMS is a disease with the greatest social impact of any disease. I think it is a major cause of social problems such as divorce and juvenile delinquency. Much marital strife is fomented by premenstrual tension. Many suffering mothers don't take care of their kids because they wake up in the morning too tired, too miserable, too irritated to feed them."

The New Approach

Based on his extensive studies, Dr. Abraham has divided PMS into four groups of symptoms:

PMS Symptoms By Groups

PMS-A	Anxiety, irritability, mood swings, nervous tension.	80 percent of women suffer from this group of symptoms.
PMS-C	Craving for sweets, dizziness, faintness, fatigue, headache, heart pounding, increased appetite.	40 percent of women suffer from this group of symptoms.
PMS-H	Abdominal bloating, breast tenderness, swelling of extemities, weight gain.	60 percent of women suffer from this group of symptoms.
PMS-D	Crying, depression, forgetfulness, insomnia.	20 percent of women suffer from this group of symptoms.

PMS-A: This subgroup includes the most commonly mentioned symptoms, and is believed to be connected to hormonal imbalance. In a double-blind crossover study there was significant improvement in PMS-A symptoms following vitamin B^6 (pyridoxine) therapy as compared to the use of a placebo. (Double-blind studies include two groups of women with the same set of symptoms. One group is given B^6 and the other group is given identical-looking tablets that are chemically inert. The results are then tabulated, and only the doctor knows which women received which tablet.)

The mechanism by which estrogen hormones influence mood is not well defined. Estrogens influence monoamine oxidase (MAO) activity. These enzymes are involved in the oxidation of epinephrine, serotonin, norepinephrine and dopamine, which are all neurotransmitters (nerve messengers). For example, epinephrine can trigger anxiety; norepinephrine, hostility; serotonin (at very high levels), drowsiness and water retention; dopamine, relaxation and mental alertness.

It is not clear yet how vitamin B^6 relieves the symptoms nor is it entirely clear how magnesium also helps alleviate tension. One theory is that vitamin B^6 stimulates the production of dopamine. It was also found that many women in the PMS-A group had severe deficiencies of minerals such as magnesium, chromium, manganese, selenium and zinc.

PMS-C: Dr. Abraham explains that the brain, which normally takes about 20 percent of the body's total energy supply, demands even more when it senses that it is under attack. The stress associated with PMS causes it to increase fuel production to meet its increased need. The extra energy has to come from glucose; this explains the craving for sweets and the fatigue, palpitations, headache and even the faintness that can follow.The liver has to process glucose from sugar. In order to do that it must have large amounts of the B-complex family of vitamins and magnesium. If a woman is eating a nutritionally sound diet, there should be adequate amounts of nutrients to meet the demand. The typical modern diet, however, does not supply the necessary nutrients, so the brain must order an emergency supply of glucose — usually from sweets. The body may demand chocolate because chocolate is a ready source of magnesium.

If stress can be avoided — marital stress, family stress, job stress, etc. — and if the patient is aware of the real need for nutrients, supplemental vitamins can supply the missing ingredients and monthly discomfort can be completely avoided.

PMS-H: This set of symptoms stems from water retention. It can result from an increase in salt intake or from the process of salt-retaining at the request of the adrenal hormone. The resulting heaviness is a real and not imaginary feeling.

PMS-D: This is perhaps the most dangerous of the menstrual states, since it encompasses thoughts of suicide, depression and withdrawals. Dr. Abraham has suggested that nutritional deficiencies can lower a woman's resistance to stress and this condition, coupled with a hormonal imbalance, may allow the dangerous state to surface.

Systems and Symptoms: A Quick Course in Recognition

Many women are told, "If you don't know whether or not you have Premenstrual Syndrome, ask your husband." Frequently husbands have said that they don't know their wives for two weeks out of every month. History shows that menstrual pain caused Queen Victoria to turn to gin and the famous nineteenth-century poet Elizabeth Barrett Browning to opium.

The chart on the following page outlines the most common aspects of PMS.

Most Common Aspects of PMS

Systems	Symptoms
Neurological	Dizziness, epilepsy, fainting spells, headache, migraine, motor coordination.
Psychological	Agression, alcoholic intervals, anger, assault/child abuse, attempted suicide, depression, drug abuse, exhaustion, frustration, irritability, lethargy, mood swings, panic, self-inflicted injury, tension, weeping.
Respiratory	Bronchitis, runny nose and/or sniffles, upper-respiratory infections.
Dermatological	Acne, boils, herpes attacks, hives, skin rashes.
Orthopedic	Backache, joint pains, stiffness.
Muscular	Abdominal pain, muscle cramps, muscle tension, water retention.
Eye	Blackness around the eyes, conjunctivitis, runny eyes.
Ear, Nose and Throat	Hoarseness, sore throat, tonsillitis.
Urological	Bloatedness, cystitis, frequent urination, urethritis, water retention.
Gastrointestinal	Abdominal swelling, food cravings, hunger pangs.
Breasts	Breast disease, breast engorgement, breast tenderness, fibrocystic breast.

Fighting PMS with Vitamins and Minerals

All minerals and vitamins are necessary for the general health and well-being of the body. However, since this is a special condition, additional supplementation, even mega-doses in some instances, may be advisable at certain times during the month.

Minerals that have been found to minimize the severity of PMS symptoms are calcium, magnesium, zinc, iron, chromium, selenium and potassium.

Calcium: Although the mineral calcium is naturally present in a number of common foods such as milk, milk products, sardines, mustard greens, turnip greens, etc., most people do not consume enough of those foods, or do not metabolize them efficiently enough to get even the Recommended Daily Allowance.

About two weeks prior to the onset of the period, the calcium level in PMS-prone individuals tends to decrease. The loss of calcium can lead to a calcium deficiency, with corresponding muscle cramps, headaches, insomnia, pelvic pain, bloating and nervousness.

A woman suffering from these symptoms, particularly pelvic pain and cramps, should take calcium in supplement form, either calcium gluconate tablets (500 mg with magnesium) or calcium citrate tablets in the desired proportion of twice as much calcium as magnesium. Vitamin D is also necessary for the uptake of calcium by the body.

Unless there is a condition that requires careful monitoring of calcium intake, an oversupply of calcium is usually excreted in the urine or with the stool. The RDA of calcium is 1,000 mg. a day; however, in the case of menstrual cramps, up to 3,000 mg a day have been used.

Magnesium: A deficiency of this mineral can cause nervousness, insomnia, muscle cramps, pelvic pain, etc. — much the same symptoms as those of calcium deficiency. These two minerals go together in a two-to-one ratio of calcium to magnesium and complement each other's activity in the body.

Nuts, soybeans and green leafy vegetables eaten raw or steamed can be sources of magnesium but most cooks do not conserve the mineral content of foods so supplementation is usually necessary.

If the woman has asked her doctor if she may take a calcium supplement, and kidney stones are no problem, then she can take half as much magnesium as calcium. If she needs 2,000 mg. of calcium to control cramps then she should take 1,000 mg of magnesium. Once the painful part of the month is over, she can lower the dosage to 1,000 mg of calcium and 500 mg of magnesium. After a few months it may not be necessary to raise the dose during those troublesome times, since the condition may adjust itself with the proper combination of diet and supplements.

Zinc: Zinc is necessary to more than fifty enzyme activities. It is found in all human tissue. Without it, RNA and DNA — the architects and builders of all the body's cells — would not develop properly. A zinc deficiency interferes with the action of the immune system since zinc is necessary to release vitamin A from its storage place in the liver. Zinc also helps to improve glucose tolerance and helps to regulate prostaglandins (hormone-like substances manufactured in many body cells) to control cramping.

To help with PMS, 30 milligrams of zinc may be taken daily and increased to 50 milligrams prior to the onset of menstruation. Irritability, depression, nervousness and headache are worsened by a zinc deficiency.

Iron: So much has been said about iron-deficiency anemia that women may be tired of hearing about it. It is, however, a fact of menstrual life. Weakness and fatigue can be overwhelming, and tiredness can easily lead to depression.

The best food sources of iron are organ meats, apricots and eggs. Many women, however, do not eat enough of these. Habit is the greatest enemy of good nutrition.

If you recognize weakness and fatigue as part of your PMS, iron — in the form of an organic compound such as ferrous gluconate or ferrous fumarate — should be taken daily. Vitamin C helps the body assimilate iron and should be taken with it.

Sometimes there is a problem with iron absorption. If supplements do not appear to counteract the feeling of weakness, the doctor should be consulted. There may be a problem with vitamin B^{12} or some other iron malabsorption situation. A severe iron deficiency needs medical treatment.

When taking separate supplements of zinc and iron, it's a good idea to take them about two hours apart. This gives each of the minerals time to be absorbed and assimilated by the body. If they are taken together, only a portion of each will be effectively assimilated.

Chromium: Carbohydrate metabolism and blood sugar levels (glucose tolerance) play a larger role in PMS than was thought previously. When sugar enters the body it triggers a release of insulin from the pancreas. This causes the blood sugar level to drop, which in turn can be the beginning of tremors, fatigue, headaches, increased appetite and a further craving for sweets. During the week prior to menses the effect of insulin on the blood sugar levels is more pronounced. Insulin is also a salt-retaining compound. Thus, the excess insulin will contribute to water retention and swelling. Chromium is a necessary trace mineral that works closely with insulin to help insure a more even balance in the bloodstream.

Potassium: A banana a day can help keep PMS away. Bananas are a good source of potassium. When a woman feels bloated, she may be retaining fluid because of a deficiency of potassium. Potassium is an electrolyte that helps to regulate water balance in the body. A deficiency may result from the use of diuretics or from a lack of intake because potassium-rich foods are not included in the diet.

Sodium is retained in the body when potassium is deficient. The result can be edema, fatigue, headache and weakness. Potassium is also necessary for normal muscle contraction, including the heart muscle.

Potassium intake may have to be increased prior to menses. The added amount is usually of little consequence to the healthy individual since excess potassium is excreted, but renal problems or cardiovascular problems may influence the dosage, so the doctor should be consulted before the use of this mineral supplement. Also, as a general rule, but specifically with potassium, make sure supplements are taken with meals to avoid stomach upset.

Selenium: This is a powerful antioxidant, particularly when combined with vitamin E, and should be taken regularly to help guard the body against internal and external radiation. In the case of PMS, selenium helps to reduce the incidence and severity of the breast tenderness symptom.

The B-complex vitamins: The diet eaten by most Americans is usually lacking in an adequate supply of the entire B-complex. Whole grains which were used to make bread and cereals — the staff of life in the past — have been stripped of most of their nutritional values, and the staff is now little more than a crutch.

B-complex vitamins are vital to all women because of their role in converting the hormone estrogen to its less active and less threatening form, estriol. If there is a deficiency of the B-complex, estrogen may build up in the breast and uterus, increasing the risk of estrogen-based cancer.

The B-vitamins particularly associated with estrogen conversion are choline, inositol, lecithin, B^6 and B^{12}. The first three are called lipotropics because they help to prevent abnormal or excessive fatty deposits in the liver. If fatty deposits are formed, the liver will not continue to deactivate the hormones that are no longer of use to the body. Again, that will mean hormone accumulation and imbalance.

Inositol, in addition to its lipotropic role, has a salutary effect on certain stressful symptoms. It has an anti-anxiety effect similar to that of a mild tranquilizer and can help to alleviate minor depressive states.

Vitamin B^6 may be the vitamin most needed by women. It appears to influence the release of two neurotransmitters in the brain called serotonin and dopamine. Neurotransmitters can serve as mood regulators and will be in short supply unless adequate vitamin B^6 is present. If there is a deficiency, the production of serotonin and dopamine may be curtailed, leading to an irrational, depressed, tense, agitated state of mind. Supplemental doses of B^6 may stabilize the situation and afford relief to the sufferer.

B^6 is a natural diuretic which can reduce fluid retention and help to relieve tension headaches and depression. It also helps to increase the body's ability to assimilate and utilize magnesium.

Although separate B-vitamins have been singled out as being of particular importance, a basic supply of all the B-vitamins must be taken as supplements before increasing the dose of any individual

B-vitamin. Like most nutritional supplements, B-vitamins work best when supplied as a team.

B-vitamins influence nerve transmission, carbohydrate metabolism and dozens of other bodily functions that directly relate to PMS. Although there are many foods that are presumed to be naturally rich in the B-vitamins, supplements are the best insurance.

Vitamin D: We can manufacture vitamin D in our bodies under the proper conditions. Those conditions are: that we are able to run around in the sun with most or all our clothes off; that no smoke, smog or air pollution interferes with the sun's rays; that the sun is at the right angle to strike our skin; and that the oil containing the vitamin has risen to the surface and is not washed off before it has had a chance to be re-absorbed and carried into the bloodstream.

So much for natural vitamin D. Calcium is dependent on vitamin D for absorption and assimilation. Therefore, those PMS symptoms that are related to a calcium deficiency are best handled by including vitamin D in the list of necessary supplements. Although the Recommended Dietary Allowance of vitamin D is 400 IU a day, some women may find they require as much as 800 IU a day to be able to control a particular set of PMS symptoms.

Vitamin E: This vitamin is utilized for normal blood circulation and has been known to ease breast tenderness. It has also been reported in *Lancet,* the British medical journal, that vitamin E has been helpful in clearing up a number of cases of fibrocystic breast disease.

Vitamin E helps to stimulate the action of the kidneys and the flow of urine, thereby reducing fluid retention. It has been known to eliminate leg cramps and to relieve pain in much the same way that aspirin does, but without the side effects.

Vitamin E is important to the adequate production and the proper metabolism of the sex hormones. It is found in high concentrations in the sex glands, the adrenals and the pituitary, all vital to the operation of the menstrual cycle. It acts to normalize these glands and to promote balance and relieve unwanted symptoms.

In its role as an antioxidant it helps to relieve stress from pollution, chemicals and drugs and from the harmful oxidation of fats in the body.

Doses of vitamin E may vary from 100 IU to 800 IU, although most people take 400 IU a day. A physician may be able to suggest the most useful amount.

Vitamin A: The normal function of vitamin A is to help maintain good vision, promote the normal, healthy development of bones and teeth, and to fight infection by strengthening the immune system and helping the body resist bacterial and viral invasion.

All endocrine glands associated with the reproductive cycle are stimulated by vitamin A. If there is insufficient vitamin A present, the glands perform at a less efficient level. A severe deficiency can result in a shutting down of production and a suspended menstrual cycle.

Vitamin A also helps to maintain the health of the cells lining the reproductive and urinary systems. Without it, problems related to the menstrual period increase tenfold. Also, since vitamin A is related to the health of the skin, acne, impetigo and hair and nail problems may indicate a need for supplementation.

Vitamin C: This vitamin is a healer in practically every condition of ill health. It builds and maintains collagen, the basis of the connective tissues that joins the body's cells, and promotes healing. Vitamin C fortifies the capillaries, helps iron into the bloodstream and prevents vitamin destruction by oxygen.

Vitamin C is concentrated in the organs and tissues that have high metabolic rates such as the brain, the adrenals, pituitary and sex glands. The adrenals are particularly sensitive to vitamin C deprivation. Although the adrenals are usually thought of as producing hormones in cases of emergency, they also secrete more than twenty steroid hormones which directly maintain the body at top efficiency. If there is not enough vitamin C present, the glands begin to shut down and hormone output is markedly decreased.

Vitamin C complex, which is a combination of vitamin C and the bioflavonoids, can be particularly useful to women during menstruation. It can help to relieve pain and irregular flow and alleviate anxiety and depression.

Vitamin C may be used in doses as high as 2,000 milligrams or more every day. Fever, infection, stress, smog, smoking, etc., increase the need for this vitamin. Medications and "the Pill" also demand additional supplies.

Other Nutritional Factors

During the weeks before menses, the effect of insulin on blood sugar is more pronounced than during the rest of the month. This can be counteracted by supplying the body with the raw materials it needs to produce a hormone called PGE-1. This hormone lessens the response of insulin to blood sugar and also decreases the central nervous system response to low blood sugar.

GLA: The raw material the body needs can be supplied by capsules of oil of Evening Primrose or by capsules of gamma-linolenic acid (GLA).

Prior to the discovery that the oil pressed from the seeds of an herb named Evening Primrose could serve as a source of essential fatty acids (called essential because they cannot be manufactured in the body but must be obtained from food or supplements), the only other known substance containing GLA (gamma linolenic acid) was mother's milk. However, nature never concentrates all of her ammunition in one form and once one vegetable or herbal source was found, investigators felt sure that they would find another one, and are now in the process of investigation.

Prostaglandins are manufactured in almost every cell in the body. They are identified by initials. It is thought that PGE2 and PGE2 Alpha are responsible for menstrual cramps, whereas PGE1 plays a beneficial role in premenstrual syndrome. In addition, there may be a lowered cholesterol level, lowered blood pressure and a strengthened immune system for the woman who fuels her body with Evening Primrose oil.

Tryptophan: The amino acid tryptophan is necessary for the production of serotonin, a brain chemical, one of the body's mood regulators. A low level of serotonin may be responsible for the "blue" mood that frequently plagues PMS victims. By supplementing the diet with tablets of L-tryptophan plus niacinamide (vitamin B^3) and pyridoxine (vitamin B^6), a higher serotonin level may be built up with a corresponding "lift" to the spirits.

Herbs: In 1875 Lydia Pinkham introduced a vegetable compound to "aid the headaches, backaches, torturing bearing down pains and dragging sensations that make women nervous and hysterical."

That preparation is still around today and women still testify to its help. The formula was an herbal combination of Jamaica dogwood, pleurisy root and licorice in an alcoholic base. Later, the homeopathic company known as Humphrey's put out another herbal formula called Humphrey's No. 11. It contained cimicifuga, pulsatilla and sepia.

For many centuries herbal medicine was the only medicine available to treat all medical conditions and it did a surprisingly good job. Herbal medications may not have the speed of modern pharmaceuticals, but they don't have the side effects, either.

Herbs are used in PMS for the following reasons: 1) to affect circulation in general; 2) to improve the quality of nutrients in the blood; 3) to improve liver function; and 4) to relieve tension and anxiety by relieving the body of excess fluid.

The following herbs have been traditionally used for "women's problems," but few medical doctors know about them and even fewer use them in their practice.

Dong quai: High in natural salycin which is the precursor to aspirin. It has been used to reduce some of the pain associated with cramping.

Black cohosh: Was an official drug listed in pharmaceutical books for nearly 100 years. Youngken's *Textbook on Herbs* says the herb is employed as a remedy for dysmenorrhea, neuralgia and tinnitus aurium (noise in the ear).

Uva ursi and buchu: Two herbs used to increase the quantity of urine expelled from the body. Also used as mild disinfectants to the urinary tract.

Other herbs that have enjoyed a reputation for aiding in relief of menstrual difficulties are arbor vitae, chamomile, elecampane, horsetail, crampbark, fo ti, passion flower, wild ginger, dandelion, couchgrass, parsley, juniper berries and pipsissewa. Herbs that have been used for nervous tension and anxiety are kava kava, valerian, scullcap, hops and chamomile.

Although not an herb, bromelain, an enzyme derived from pineapple, is also helpful for PMS patients because of its anti-inflammatory effects.

It is also important to eliminate certain substances from the body by eliminating them from the diet. Salt, alcohol and caffeine can cause irritability and breast tenderness. Nicotine (either from smoking or being in the same area as a smoker) restricts circulation. Overindulgence in red meat, fats and dairy products can interfere with magnesium absorption. Salt causes water retention. White flour, chocolate and alcohol potentiate the symptoms of PMS.

It is advisable to eat substantial amounts of unrefined complex carbohydrates. These include potatoes, wholegrain breads, cereals and pasta, green leafy vegetables, beans, peas, lentils and nuts. Fish and poultry should be substituted for red meats. Eat small, frequent meals or snacks to keep blood sugar at a normal level.

The natural ways to beat PMS are quite effective, but a word of caution is in order to women who want to start to use them. Diet and supplements do not work as fast as prescription or over-the-counter drugs. Allow six months of consistent nutritional therapy to see results; your reward will be freedom from PMS for the rest of your reproductive years.

References

Abraham, G.E. "Nutritional Factors in the Etiology of the Premenstrual Tension Syndrome." *The Journal of Reproductive Medicine*, Vol. 28, No. 7.

A Barefoot Doctor's Manual: The American Translation of the Official Chinese Paramedical Manual. Philadelphia: Running Press, 1977.

Brewer, J.I. *Textbook of Gynecology*. Baltimore: Williams and Wilkins, 1962.

Budoff, P.W. *No More Menstrual Cramps and Other Good News.* New York: G.P. Putnam & Sons, 1980.

Goldbeck, N. *How to Cope with Menstrual Problems: A Wholistic Approach.* New Canaan, Conn.: Keats Publishing, Inc., 1983.

Lauersen, N.H., and Stukane, E. *Premenstrual Syndrome and You.* New York: Simon & Schuster, 1983.

Novak, E., and Novak, E.R. *Textbook of Gynecology*. Baltimore:

Williams and Wilkins, 1952.

Sampson, G.A. "Premenstrual Syndrome: A Double-Blind Controlled Trial of Progesterone and Placebo." *British Journal of Psychiatry* 135: 209-215.

Stokes, J., and Mendels, J. "Pyridoxine and Premenstrual Tension."

Lancet I: 1177-78.

PART III

CAUTION: IF YOU ARE TAKING PRESCRIPTION DRUGS THE FOOD YOU EAT MAY BE DANGEROUS TO YOUR HEALTH

You might be swallowing more than the doctor ordered if you mix prescription drugs with other medications, alcohol, over-the-counter products or even the wrong foods warns "FDA Consumer."

Your doctor or pharmacist cannot follow you to the dinner table or to the general store. Drug labeling, informed health professionals and this chapter can be helpful to you.

SIDE EFFECTS OF "SAFE" DRUGS

Drug	Possible Side Effects
Acne medications	Stinging, burning, itching, swelling, dryness, bleaching of hair; dark brown scale on dark-skinned people.
Antacids	Constipation, acid rebound, loss of appetite, diarrhea, kidney stones.
Antidiarrheals	Dependence, tiredness, bacterial infections, gastric pain, bloating, constipation.
Antihistamine	Fatigue, upset stomach, blurred vision, nausea, constipation, diarrhea.
Appetite suppressants	Nervousness, insomnia, restlessness, nausea, headache, high blood pressure, hallucinations, anxiety.
Cough medicines	Thickened mucus, nausea, constipation, dependence, drowsiness, light-headedness, allergic reaction, itching, heart palpitations, flushing, blurred vision, upset stomach.
Diuretics	Nausea, headache, drowsiness, mental confusion, hyperventilation.
Hemorrhoid creams	High blood pressure, heart arrhythmia, nervousness, insomnia, aggravated hyperthyroidism, skin irritation.
Laxatives	Abdominal discomfort, faintness, rectal burning, cramps, dependence, skin rashes, poor nutrient absorption, intestinal obstruction, dehydration, diarrhea.
Nasal decongestants	Nasal irritation; decreased effectivness of decongestants, resulting in addiction.
Pain-relief pills	Skin reactions, vomiting, heartburn, gastric distress and bleeding, nausea, iron deficiency anemia, gastric ulcers, blood in stools, aggravated asthma.
Sleep aids	Excitation, dizziness, ringing in ears, blurred vision, gastrointestinal disturbances, dry mouth, dependence.

14

FOOD AND DRUG INTERACTION MAY BE HARMFUL TO YOUR HEALTH

Introduction

What is meant by a Food — Drug Interaction?

Very simply stated, it means that the food you eat and the liquids you drink can alter the effect of the drug you are taking.

Why is this important?

If there is an interaction, it can make the drug have a greater or lesser effect.

For example:

Fruit juices, vegetable juices, colas and other sodas and wines, are acid in nature and will reduce the strength of antibiotics like penicillin, ampicillin and erythromycin.

On the other hand, if you are taking a medication that contains iron, it would be best to take it with a fruit juice that contains a high amount of vitamin C because vitamin C aids the absorption and assimilation of iron in the stomach.

This part of the book deals with some of the most common food-drug interactions but not with all of them. It is meant strictly for information and not for self-diagnosis or treatment. You must check with your doctor for complete information about the prescription drug you are taking and any possible food-drug interaction. Do not discontinue any medication or avoid any particular food without first consulting him or her.

In general, if you must avoid any food or groups of foods, it may be appropriate to use a multi-vitamin/mineral supplement to insure a constant supply of any nutrient that may be lost.

You May Be Swallowing More Than the Doctor Ordered

You might be setting yourself up for more side effects than the doctor told you of if you mix prescription drugs with other medications, over-the-counter remedies, alcohol, cigarettes, or even the wrong foods.

Side effects can be mild, such as a slight rash, headache, nausea or drowsiness, to severe, which can include prolonged vomiting, bleeding, weakness, impaired vision or hearing, loss of key nutrients, a medical crisis or — in rare instances — death.

When two drugs with the same impact are consumed together, the results can be greater than anticipated. A situation known as potentiation, which can be helpful or dangerous depending on the medication, can develop.

Would it occur to you not to swallow a tetracycline capsule with a glass of milk? Or to avoid aged cheese or a glass of Chianti wine if you are taking a certain medicine to fight hypertension? Would you think to eat more leafy green vegetables if you are on the Pill?

Probably not.

Yet the effects the food and drugs have on each other can often determine whether the medication will do its job and whether your body gets the nutrients it needs.

The extent of the interaction between foods and drugs is influenced by a number of factors.

- Drug dosage
- Individuals' age and weight
- General physical condition
- General nutritional condition
- Specific medical condition

As a general rule, the presence of food in the stomach and the intestines can drastically slow the drug's travel through the intestinal tract to the body area where it is needed.

Some foods contain natural and added chemicals that can react with the prescribed medication to make it virtually useless.

Some of these reactions can be dangerous enough to make a telephone call to the doctor absolutely vital.

One major way food affects drugs is by enhancing or impeding absorption of the drug into the bloodstream.

Fatty foods will speed up the action of the drug griseofulvin, a medication used internally to help fight fungus infections, especially of the nails. In this situation, eating fatty foods will be a help in the battle against ringworm and other fungus infections.

More often this is not the case. Foods usually interfere with absorption of the drug, as with tetracycline and milk. Dairy products contain varying amounts of calcium, and calcium interferes with the absorption of tetracycline, but before this was known, doctors told their patients to take this antibiotic with a glass of milk because it was thought the milk would help prevent irritation of the stomach lining. Instead, it prevented the full activity of the antibiotic!

As a general rule, you shouldn't take prescription drugs with acid fruit, vegetable juice, soda (Coke, Pepsi, Seven-Up, Root Beer, etc.) unless you first ask your doctor or pharmacist if there will be any problems. The reason is the chance of excess acidity.

Why Worry About The Acidity?

Some drugs are designed to resist the acid of the stomach and dissolve lower down in the intestinal tract. The excess acid will eat away the coating on the drug and cause it to dissolve more quickly in an area where it will not be readily absorbed.

Excessive consumption of foods containing vitamin K can interfere with the effectiveness of drugs involved in the clotting process. When *anticoagulants* are prescribed (drugs that help prevent clotting) liver and green leafy vegetables should be avoided with your doctor's agreement.

To prevent possible reactions between MAO inhibiting drugs and food, the following should be avoided:

- Aged and fermented foods
- Pickled herring
- Salami and pepperoni

- Sharp or aged cheese
- Yogurt and sour cream
- Beef and chicken livers
- Fava beans
- Canned figs
- Bananas and avocados
- Soy sauce
- Beer, Chianti wine, Sherry and other wines in large amounts

Also, although not specifically dangerous to all people, there have been reported cases of adverse reactions with cola beverages, chocolate and even raisins.

The reason for the avoidance of certain foods, even though it may be considered a hardship, is the danger of severe headaches, brain hemorrhage and, in extreme cases, death because of the reaction between the MAO inhibitor drugs and a substance in the mentioned foods called *Tyramine*.

And now to mention alcohol.

Even though the FDA doesn't recognize alcohol as a drug, it is one.

Alcohol does not mix well with other drugs. When it is combined with antihistamines, antidepressants or tranquilizers it can cause excessive drowsiness. If you are driving a car, operating heavy machinery or conducting any task that requires you to be alert, the combination can be dangerous.

Alcohol also does not mix with other drugs such as antibiotics, anticoagulants, antidiabetic drugs, high blood pressure drugs or sedatives. And just because you can buy something without a prescription doesn't make it alcohol-safe. As a general rule, don't take any type of medication with alcohol.

Cigarettes can also interfere with your prescription. Smoking can break down theophylline (drug used to help asthmatics), pentazocine (pain killer), tranquilizers, analgesics and antidepressants. As a result, smokers may need larger doses of these medications.

Smoking can also alter the results on diagnostic tests such as red and white blood cell counts and blood clotting time determination.

Drug interactions can also cause false readings on laboratory tests. If you take a lot of laxatives, it will have an effect on tests for calcium or bone metabolism. Penicillin can lead to a false reading of urine protein, indicating kidney disease to be present when it is not. An excessive amount of vitamin C can alter results in urinary glucose tests for diabetes.

Just as some drugs are affected by foods, so can some drugs interfere with your body's ability to convert those nutrients into a usable form — and flush those nutrients out before they've done their real job.

Colchicine and mineral oil can prevent the absorption of nutrients from the bowel. Hydralazine and the anti-tuberculosis drug INH can deplete the body's supplies of vitamin B^6 by inhibiting production of an enzyme necessary to convert the food vitamin into a form that is usable by the body.

Anticonvulsant drugs that are used to help control epilepsy can lead to deficiencies of folic acid and vitamin D because they increase the loss of these nutrients from the body.

Neomycin, colchicine and oral antidiabetic agents can impair the absorption of vitamin B^{12}.

"Water pills" can lead to serious potassium depletion, as most patients know, because their doctors recommend adding tomatoes, oranges, dried apricots, cantaloupes, figs, raisins, bananas, prunes, potatoes, sweet potatoes and winter squash to the diet for the potassium content.

Because of these potential side effects, you should tell your doctor about any allergies you have before he or she prescribes a medication. Tell him or her about any prescription drugs or OTC products you're fond of taking and any condition you are now being treated for by another physician. Also, whether you have any existing diabetes or liver problems and whether or not you smoke and/or drink.

Medications should correct existing problems, not create new ones!

What Do Your Doctor's Directions Mean?

"Take 4 times a day."

Is that every six hours — that's 4 times a day?

Do I get up during the night?

What if the doctor says, "take before meals."

Is it right before meals, one hour before meals, or what?

The same goes for after meals.

Take with a liquid.

Is that to mean water, beer, soda, milk, a martini?????

And, how much liquid? A glass, two glasses or just a swallow?

IF THE DIRECTIONS ARE NOT CLEAR TO YOU, ASK YOUR DOCTOR TO SPELL IT OUT AND KEEP ASKING UNTIL YOU ARE SURE YOU UNDERSTAND.

Drugs That Are Usually Taken With Food Unless Instructed Otherwise By Your Doctor

Aldactazide
Aldactone
Aldoril
Amesec
Aminodur
APC's
Apresazide
Apresoline
Aristocort
Artane
Aspirin
Azolid
Bronkotabs
Brondecon
Butagesic
Butazolidin
Celestone
Chlorothiazide
Colace
Cortisone
Darvon Compound
Decagesic
Delta Cortef
Deltasone
Dialose
Dilantin
Di-Phen
Diupres
Diuril
Diphenyl
Diphenylan
Doxycycline
Dralserp
Dralzine
Dyazide
Edecrin
Elixophyllin
Emprazil
Enduron
Erythromycin
Esidrix
Esimil
Flagyl
Ferrous Sulfate
Feosol

Furadantin
Furalan
Furaloid
Griseofulvin
Hexadrol
Hydralazine
Hydrochlorothiazide
Hydrodiuril
Hydropres
Hygrotin
Indocin
Indomethacin
Inderal
Lexor
Lithium
Lopressor
Macrodantin
Malcogesic
Marax
Medrol
Metroprolol
Motrin
Neggram
Nitrex
Nitrofor
Nitrofurantoin
Oretic
Oxalid
Parfuran
Pediamycin
Percodan
Phenbutazone
Ponstel
Propoxyphene
Propranolol
Prednisolone
Prednisone
Quadrinal
Quibron
Quinidine
Reserpine
Rauzide
Regroton
Renese-R
Salutensin
Sandril
Ser-Ap-Es
Serpasil
Spironolactone
Sterazolidin
Tandearil
Tedral
Trantoin
Tramterene
Unipres
Urotoin
Vibramycin

NOTE: This is not a complete listing of all of the drugs that should be taken with food. Your doctor is the final word on how it should be taken. Also, although a drug should be taken with food, there are certain foods that may cause side effects when taken with certain drugs. Again, make sure you ask your doctor for specific instructions.

Drugs Better Taken One Hour Before Meals Or Two Hours After Meals Unless Instructed Otherwise By Your Doctor

Ampicillin	Lincocin	Probantheline
Amoxicillin	Oxytetracycline	Prostaphlin
Declomycin	Penicillamine	Rifampin
Erythromycin	Penicillin G	TAO
Erythromycin Stearate	Penicillin V	Tegopen
Isoniazid	Penicillin V K	Tetracycline
Levadopa	Pentaerythritol Tetranitrate	Unipen

NOTE: This is not a complete listing and many of the drugs on the list appear under other names. The only way to be sure is to check with your doctor or your pharmacist.

15

CLASSES OF DRUGS AND FOODS TO AVOID WHEN TAKING THEM

Antibiotics

Drug or Class of Drugs

Tetracycline Antibiotics
Achromycin
Aureomycin
Bristacycline
Cyclopar
Declomycin
Panmycin
Rondomycin
Sumycin
Terramycin
Tetra-Bid
Tetrachel
Tetracyn
Tetrex

NOTE: Exceptions — Doxychel, Vibramycin, Vibratabs, Minocin.

Foods to be Avoided During Course of Treatment

Take the medication one hour before ingesting milk or milk products or two hours after ingesting milk or milk products.

Reason

The infection may not be controlled properly.

Anticoagulants

Drug or Class of Drugs

Anticoagulants —	Athrombin - K
	Coufarin
	Coumadin
	Dicumarol
	Hedulin
	Miradon
	Panwarfin

Usual Use

To prevent clotting of blood.

Foods to be avoided During Course of Treatment

Asparagus	Liver
Broccoli	Lettuce
Brussels sprouts	Onions
Cabbage	Peas
Cauliflower	Spinach
Garlic	Turnip greens
Kale	Watercress
	Other leafy green vegetables

Reason

The effect of the anticoagulant may be decreased and blood may clot despite the treatment.

NOTE: If the doctor agrees, small amounts of these foods may be eaten because they contain important nutrients. If they must be avoided altogether, supplements are recommended. Read the label carefully to make sure the supplement you get does not contain vitamin K.

Antidepressants

Drug or Class of Drugs

Parnate
Marplan
Nardil
Eutonyl

Usual Use

Antidepressant

Foods to be Avoided During Course of Treatment

Avocados
Baked potatoes
Bananas
Beer
Bologna
Brie
Broad beans
Caviar
Cheeses
Chicken livers
Chocolate
Coffee
Colas
Canned figs
Meat tenderizers
Nuts
Pickled Herring
Raspberries
Salami
Sauerkraut
Sour cream
Soy sauce
Wines
Yeast
Yogurt

Reason

If the drug is combined with certain foods, it can cause a marked rise in blood pressure, with all the problems that can bring.

NOTE: Your doctor will give you a complete list of foods that should be avoided when using this type of medication. If dining at a friend's house, be sure to show him or her the list to see if you can or cannot eat some of the foods on the menu.

Antifungal Drugs

Drugs or Class of Drugs

Griseofulvin
Fulvicin P/G U/F
Grifulvin V
Grisactin
Gris - PEG

Usual Use

To combat fungal infections of the hair, nails and skin.

Foods to be Taken During Course of Treatment

Avocados
Butter
Cream
Cakes
Beef
Fried Foods

Reason

The beneficial effect of the drug is increased when taken with fatty foods. This drug should be taken with meals.

Asthma Drugs

Drug or Class of Drugs

Asthma drugs containing theophylline

Accurbron
Amesec
Asbron
Brondecon
Bronkodyl
Choledyl
Dilor
Elixicon
Elixohyllin
Lufyllin
Marax
Mudrane
Quibron
Quibron-T
Respbid
Somophyllin
Sustaire
Tedral SA
Theobid
Theodur
Theolair
Theophyl

Usual Use

To make breathing easier for asthmatics by opening lung air passages.

Foods to be Avoided During Treatment

Any charcoal-broiled meats

Reason

The effects of the drug may be decreased and the asthma condition may not be controlled as effectively.

Asthma Drugs (Continued)

Drug or Class of Drugs

Asthma Drugs containing theophylline

Usual Use

To make breathing easier for asthmatics by opening lung air passages.

Foods to be Avoided During Course of Treatment

Coffee

Tea

Colas or other caffeine-containing soft drinks

Chocolate

Cocoa

Any other medication or over-the-counter products that contain caffeine.

Reason

The effects can be increased so that side effects may be noted such as: nausea, dizziness, headache, irritability, insomnia, heartbeat irregularities.

Bisacodyl Laxatives

Drug or Class of Drugs

Bisacodyl Laxatives — Bical
Biscolax
Dulcolax
Theralax
Ulcolax
Vacterol

Usual Use

Laxative

Foods to be Avoided During Course of Treatment

These products should not be taken with milk or within one hour of taking milk or antacids.

Reason

The medicine is coated with an enteric compound. An alkaline environment may cause the drug to dissolve in the wrong area, giving you gastritis.

Cardiac Drugs

Drug or Class of Drugs

Quinidine
Quinaglute
Quinidex
Quinora
Duraquin
Cardioquin

Usual Use

To restore irregular heart beats to normal rhythm.

Foods to be Avoided During Course of Treatment

Almonds
Buttermilk

Chestnuts
Orange Juice
Grapefruit Juice
Lemon Juice
Milk
Cream
Alkaline Fruit (except plums, prunes, cranberries)
Vegetables (except lentils, corn)

Reason

The effect of Quinidine can result in possible side effects such as headache, ringing in the ears, palpitations, or heart beat irregularities when these foods are eaten during the course of your treatment.

Heart Drugs #2

Drug or Class of Drugs

Digoxin
Lanoxin

Usual Use

USED IN CASES OF CONGESTIVE HEART FAILURE AND TO RESTORE IRREGULAR HEARTBEAT TO A NORMAL RHYTHM.

Foods to be Avoided During Course of Treatment

High fiber foods should be eaten at least one hour before taking medication because the effect of the medication may be decreased.

Prunes or prune juice
Oat or Wheat Bran
Whole wheat foods
Raw vegetables
Fruits
Cooked leafy vegetables

NOTE: Because these foods are important to the diet, medication should be taken one hour before or two hours after eating them, but they should not be avoided altogether unless your doctor advises this.

Heart Drugs #2 (Continued)

Drug or Class of Drugs

All Digitalis-Containing Heart Drugs

Crystodigin	Lanoxin
Digifortis	Purodigin

Usual Use

Use in cases of congestive heart failure and to restore irregular heartbeat to a normal rhythym.

Foods to be Avoided During Course of Treatment

Natural licorice in capsule form or in candy form.

Synthetic licorice can be used.

Reason

The strength of the drug may be increased with possible side effects such as loss of energy, loss of appetite, nausea, headache, confusion, visual disturbances and heartbeat irregularities.

Drugs For Mental Disorders

Drugs or Class of Drugs

Lithium
Eskalith
Lithane
Lithonate
Lithobid
Litho-tabs
Lithonate - S

Usual Use

Mental disorders

Foods to be Avoided During Course of Treatment

Low salt diet increases the effect of lithium.

High salt diet decreases the effect of lithium.

Reason

Too little salt can cause dizziness, dry mouth, weakness, confusion, loss of appetite, loss of energy, nausea, slurred speech, loss of coordination.

Too much salt will interfere with the proper action of the drug.

The doctor must advise on the correct salt content since many foods contain salt without listing it or the amount on the label.

Leg Cramp Drugs

Drug or Class of Drugs

Quinine

Quinamm

Coco-Quinine

Quine

Usual Use

Malaria, nighttime leg cramps.

Foods to be Avoided During Course of Treatment

Almonds	Chestnuts
Buttermilk	Milk
Orange Juice	Cream
Grapefruit Juice	Alkaline Fruit (except plums, prunes, cranberries)
Lemon Juice	Vegetables (except lentils, corn)

Reason

The effect of the drug may be increased, with possible side effects such as dizziness, headache, ringing in the ears, or visual disturbance.

Parkinson's Disease

Drug or Class of Drugs

Levodopa
Dopar
Laradopa
Sinemet

Usual Use

Control the tremors of Parkinson's Disease.

Foods to be Avoided During Course of Treatment

Avocados	Molasses
Bacon	Navy beans
Brewer's Yeast	Oatmeal
Bran products	Pork
Beef kidney	Soybeans
Beef liver	Split peas
Dry skim milk	Sweet potatoes
Fresh salmon	Tuna
Kidney beans	Walnuts
Lentils	Wheat germ
Lima beans	Yams

NOTE: Vitamin B^6 (pyridoxine) must be avoided. Many vitamin combinations contain this important vitamin. You may have to take mineral supplements separately and vitamins individually to avoid the B^6.

Reason

The effect of the medication may be decreased and the condition will not be controlled properly.

Thyroid Drugs

Drug or Class of Drugs

Thyroid
Cytomel
Euthroid
Levothroid
Proloid
Synthroid
Thyrar
Thyrolar

Usual Use

Prescribed to correct insufficient function of the thyroid.

Foods to be Avoided During Course of Treatment

Asparagus
Broccoli
Brussels Sprouts
Cabbage
Kale
Lettuce
Peas
Spinach
Turnip greens
Other green leafy vegetables

Reason

The effect of the medication may be minimized. Avoid green leafy vegetables or eat only tiny portions.

Urinary Antiseptics

Drug or Class of Drugs

Hiprex
Mandelamine
Methenamine
Urex

Usual Use

Urinary antiseptic to combat urinary tract infections

Foods to be Avoided During Course of Treatment

Almonds
Buttermilk
Chestnuts
Orange Juice
Grapefruit Juice
Lemon Juice
Milk
Cream
Alkaline Fruit (except plums, prunes, cranberries)
Vegetables (except lentils, corn)

Reason

The effect of the drug may be decreased.

Some Cautions and Examples of Side Effects Most Doctors Don't Think About — Unless You Ask Them!

It's your body.

You have to be on the lookout for products containing alcohol or aspirin if you're taking antidiabetic drugs such as:

- Acetohexamide (Dymelor)
- Chlorpropamide (Diabinese)
- Insulin
- Tolbutamide (Orinase)
- Tolazamide (Tolinase)
- or any other antidiabetic drug

You have to be on the lookout for products containing alcohol or aspirin. Alcohol can either increase or lower your blood sugar level. Aspirin, in combination with your medication, can lower your blood sugar level.

You're aware enough not to drink alcoholic beverages and you are also aware enough to avoid Bayer aspirin. But what about all of the following over-the-counter products which contain either alcohol or aspirin?

- Alka Seltzer
- Anacin
- Bufferin
- Aspergum
- Cough syrups like Cheracol and Cheracol D, Cosanyl-DM, Robitussin
- Dristan
- Ecotrin
- Empirin
- Excedrin
- Measurin
- Midol
- Neo-Synephrine
- Novahistine
- Nyquil
- Pamprin
- Pepto Bismol
- Triaminic
- Vicks Formula 44 or 44D

You must ask questions and read labels.

If you're taking anticoagulants you should also avoid any of the aspirin-containing products because they can increase the activity of your medication and lead to excessive bleeding.

If you are taking steroids on prescription such as:

- Betamethasone
- Cortisone
- Dexamethasone
- Flurocortisone

- Hydrocortisone
- Methylproednisolone
- Prednisolone
- Prednisone
- Triamcinolone

Avoid alcohol and aspirin products. If mixed, there is increased potential for nausea, vomiting or damage to your stomach lining.

Diuretics mixed with alcohol or decongestant cold remedies could cause dizziness and decreased mental alertness.

Antihypertensives mixed with alcohol can cause severe drowsiness and a loss of mental acuity.

Antihypertensive drugs with cough or cold remedies which contain a decongestant could increase or decrease your blood pressure.

Antianxiety or sedative drugs with alcohol can result in severe dizziness, nausea and decrease mental acuity.

If mixed with OTC products containing alcohol (even a little), it could result in depression of your central nervous system.

When you are taking any type of prescription drug, you are vulnerable to side reactions from the drug and from its combination with anything else you put into your mouth. Since you are in a vulnerable position you must defend yourself by asking questions. Before you take any OTC product internally, ask your doctor or your pharmacist if the pharmacist is aware of all the medications you are taking.

If you are a member of AARP, they have issued a comprehensive PRESCRIPTION DRUG HANDBOOK with expert information on the safe and effective use of the medicines most frequently prescribed for persons 50 and over. It is also available in some bookstores.

If the information you are seeking is not listed, don't give up. Ask your health professional.

Smoking and Medication — Some Particulars

Maybe your smoking habit is the reason you have to take prescription drugs now and maybe not. But, either way, if you're still smoking you can alter the effect your prescription drug is having on your body.

Here are just a few of the major effects that have been reported:

DRUG	EFFECT
Acetaminophen	Smokers have to take higher doses.
Antidepressants	Smokers have to take higher doses.
Benzodiazepine	Reduced effectiveness.
Caffeine	Less central nervous system stimulation.
Glutethimide	Smokers get increased effect.
Pentazocine	Larger maintenance doses may be needed.
Phenobarbital	Reduced effectiveness.
Phenothiazine	Reduced effectiveness.
Phenylbutazone	Reduced effectiveness.
Propoxyphene	Reduced effectiveness.
Propanolol	Reduced effectiveness.
Theophylline	Reduced effectiveness.

It is possible that, even if you don't smoke but are habitually in a smoky atmosphere, similar effects can be manifested.

Drugs that Interfere with Your Nutrition

We all need vitamins, minerals, trace minerals, accessory nutrients etc. The lack of one nutrient can effect the status of all of the nutrients in the body. The body requires over 40 different essential nutrients. If your medication interferes with any nutrient, it is reasonable to assume that supplementation can help to restore the body's supplies — providing you are aware of what you may be missing!

The following table illustrates *some* but not all drug reactions which may interfere with your nutritional state.

This is not a complete guide since there are thousands of drugs and not all reactions have been catalogued. Also, new drugs come out every year.

Your doctor and your pharmacist are your best guides.

The information in the listing and in the rest of this book is for educational purposes and not intended for self treatment. Do not discontinue any prescribed medication without the advice of your doctor. If your health professional suggests that nutritional supplements could be helpful, take your medication and your supplements about two hours apart.

These Drugs May Cause Nutrient Depletion

Drugs or Drug Class	Nutrients Depleted
Anorectic Agents (including amphetamines)	$B\text{-}^{12}$, C, Potassium
Antacids	A, B^1, B^2, B^{12}, D, Folic Acid, Iron, Phosphates
Antibiotics	A, B^{12}, C, E, K, Biotin, Calcium, Iron, Magnesium, Potassium
Anticonvulsants	B^2, B^{12}, C, D, K, Folic Acid, Calcium, Magnesium
Antidiabetics (Oral)	B^2, B^{12}, C, D, Folic Acid
Antituberculosis Drugs	B^6, B^{12}, E, Folic Acid, Iron
Aspirin (Salicylates)	B^6, B^{12}, C, E, K, Folic Acid, Iron (by GI blood loss)
Cardiac Glycosides	D, Calcium, Magnesium
Chelators	Copper, Iron, Magnesium, Zinc
Cholestyramine	A, B^{12}, D, E, Folic Acid, K, Iron, Potassium
Clofibrate	A, B^{12}, Iron, K
Colchicine	B^{12}
Contraceptive Steroids (oral)	B^1, B^2, B^6, B^{12}, C, E, Folic Acid, Niacin
Corticosteroids	B^2, C, D, Niacin, Zinc
Cycloserine	B^{12}, Folic Acid, K, Calcium, Magnesium

Drugs or Drug Class	Nutrients Depleted
Digitalis	B^1
Diuretics(check particular ones)	B^1, B^{12}, D, Folic Acid, Calcium (not Thiazides), Magnesium, Potassium, Zinc
Glucocorticoids	B^2, C, D, Niacin, Calcium, Potassium, Zinc
Glutethimide	D
Hydralazine	B^6
Irritant Cathartics	D
Isoniazea	B^6, Niacin
Laxatives	A, B^2, B^{12}, D, Folic Acid, Iron, Phosphate, Calcium and Potassium for Laxative Abuse
Methotrexate	Folic Acid
Mineral Oil	A, D, E, K
Muscle Relaxers	B^2, B^{12}, C, D, Folic Acid
Neomycin	A, B^2, B^6, B^{12}, Iron
Penicillamine	B^6, Copper, Zinc
Potassium Chloride	B^{12}
Pyrimethamine	Folic Acid
Sulfasalazine	Folic Acid
Tetracycline	C
Triamterene	Folic Acid
Trifluoperazine	B^{12}
Trimethoprim	Folic Acid

A LAST-MINUTE GIFT

How To Beat One of the Greatest Youth Robbers of Them All — Insomnia

It's at night that the body rebuilds cells destroyed during the day, makes new tissues and encourages the restructuring of neurotransmitters.

Night is recuperation time, the sleep that knits the ravelled sleeves . . . but only if you fall asleep quickly and sleep soundly. A bad night's sleep can rob you of energy and youth, make you feel and look older.

Egyptian Proverb

The worst things:
To want for one who comes not,
To try to please and please not,
To be in bed and sleep not.

What Is Sleep and Why Do We Sleep?

Very little is known about sleep although there have been volumes written about it. We know that sleep is one of life's essentials. If we didn't sleep we couldn't survive. In general, we say that, in the sleeping state, the brain regenerates its fund of nerve energy and marshals other vital factors, some known and some still unknown to us.

So, let's explore the realm of sleep and how to insure that its effects benefit your longevity.

What Do We Mean When We Say "A Good Night's Sleep?"

When we sleep well, we're able to think, work, and handle stress better. When we sleep badly or not at all, we feel tired, stressed, have difficulty solving big and little problems, and just can't enjoy life.

Psychologists label sleep a normal bodily function, and when it's disturbed, the balance of all body systems is also disturbed. How long and how well we sleep affects not only our attitudes, but our immune system too. While we sleep and the other body systems slow to a crawl, the immune system regenerates itself, repairing the organs and tissues that have to be in top shape to protect the body. Anyone lacking sleep for a length of time would get physically sick or mentally sick.

How Long A Length Of Time?

That varies from person to person. What is recommended is to get as much sleep as you need to be wide-awake and bright-eyed. Most people need from seven to nine hours of sleep according to Richard Allen, Ph.D., A.C.P., a psychologist at Johns Hopkins Sleep Disorder Center in Baltimore, Maryland. However, most people try to cut their sleep time a little shorter than they should.

If I Have Trouble Falling Asleep, Should I Try Harder?

Usually that won't help. If you are having trouble falling asleep, or if your sleep has been interrupted, it may be best to get out of bed and even go out of the bedroom into another room. Watch television, read a book, crochet, or try a warm, not hot, bath. Soon you'll be relaxed enough to go back to bed and sleep.

I Do Fall Asleep But It Sometimes Takes Hours.

Maybe you're going to bed too early in the evening. If you go to bed before you are sleepy, even if you do manage to put yourself to sleep, you can have a disturbed rest rather than a restful sleep. If you go to sleep because the clock says you should be sleepy, you could wake up without feeling refreshed. Go to sleep when you feel sleepy. That can be earlier or later than what your clock says.

When I was a kid I fell asleep as soon as my head hit the pillow. Now I can't sleep as well as I used to.

Everything changes, including sleep patterns. About the age of fifty, most people's sleep patterns change as a result of aging or life-style shift. The children are gone, your job is tedious, stress is greater or lesser. The old sleep schedule you set for yourself may have changed and you go to bed too early or too late. Maybe you're planning to retire and your mind is too active at night as you try to figure if you'll have enough income. What can you do? Once you're aware of the cause, you will probably come up with the solution.

In That Case, Since I'm Older, Can I Get Along With Less Sleep And Not Feel It?

Sleep patterns change but sleep needs do not show a significant decrease as we age. Unless there are medical reasons to spend more time in a sleep-recuperative mode, or if you're taking naps in the afternoon, you still need your regular eight to nine hours of satisfying sleep at night.

Cigarettes Usually Relax Me At Work, Will They Help Me To Fall Asleep At Night?

The nicotine in cigarettes is actually a stimulant to your nervous system and will interfere with your ability to fall asleep. The reason you think it relaxes you during the day while you're on the job is because you are getting your "nicotine fix." Your body says it's hungry for nicotine and you satisfy the urge. Try not smoking at all for better health, or try not to smoke for one hour before you try to sleep.

I Wake Up A Number Of Times During The Night. How Can I Stop?

A baby will sleep through a thunderstorm. As you get older, sleep becomes more fragmented and you sleep less deeply and less efficiently. The lighter sleep patterns can make you more aware of shifting lights, noises, and even odors. Try to insure an even darkness and quiet. Keep the temperature at a level that helps you sleep best. Too much heat or cold will awaken you. Make the conditions as comfortable as you can but if you do wake up too early, don't brood about it. Get up and start your day a little earlier.

Can Naps Help Insomnia?

Yes and no. If you're not getting enough sleep at night, a nap during the day can help you get some sleep time. But, some people who nap during the day can't sleep at night. Try a nap and see which group you fit into.

I Don't Dream. Is That Why I Don't Feel Rested?

You do dream . . . you just don't remember your dreams. Everyone dreams, and in full color! The people who remember black and white dreams are focusing on the dream content even if the dream was a technicolor beauty. Nightmares can interfere with restful, productive sleep, but outside of that, dreams are an exciting part of life. If dreams are disturbing on a regular basis, it might be best to discuss the situation with a health counselor.

What About Snoring?

If it's your snoring, it's trivial. If it's your spouse's snoring . . . it's terrible.

In the latter case, get separate bedrooms.

Seriously, snoring is always a sign of impaired breathing during sleep. Light snoring is trivial and may even lull the listener to sleep. Heavy snoring, followed by a feeling of extreme tiredness the following day, can be a sign of a sleep disorder called sleep apnea. This is a condition in which the sleeper repeatedly stops breathing while asleep. Although anyone can experience breathing irregularities once in a while, the person suffering from sleep apnea may stop breathing from ten to 90 seconds. This situation can occur several hundred times a night without the sufferer being aware of the situation.

Sleep apnea is most frequently found in middle-aged overweight men, but can also afflict men or women of any age.

People suffering from this condition can experience irregular breathing for up to 70 percent of their total night's sleep. The cause can be a deviated septum, polyps, large adenoids, tonsils, or a host of other problems. Although just about everyone has experienced an odd bout of insomnia, for an estimated 50 to 100 million Americans it's a regular occurrence. And for 20 to 40 million of them, the condition is chronic and disrupts their health. Many people suffer outright sleeping disorders.

Dr. William Dement, professor of psychiatry at Stamford University and chairman of the National Commission on Sleep Disorder Research, considers sleep deprivation to be a national epidemic. Tests show the average American adult is almost pathologically sleepy. Observations from traffic engineers and from the television industry indicate that sleep patterns are changing in this country.

There are two reasons:

- People with sleep illnesses.
- People who are "sleep cheating."

"Sleep cheats" are not insomniacs. They can go to bed and fall asleep, but won't. They won't miss the late television show; can't break away from the poker game; can't stop talking and go to bed.

Millions of people stay up late out of habit. Many feel that the late evening hours are the only ones they can call their own. Tired housewives who have put their children to bed feel that now, finally, they're entitled to a little time to themselves.

The candle is burning at both ends!

There are other reasons for less sleep hours. The increasing number of two-job couples means they have to run errands and do chores before going to work. The average age of the population is increasing. Societal changes favor less sleep. It's a go-go world, open 24 hours a day. If you don't bank during the day, do it at night. Shop at night, watch the Home Shopping station on TV and buy presents at night. Many late stayer-uppers hang on simply because they're dissatisfied with what they've accomplished during the day. We've made Gods out of the businessman who talks about working so hard that he gets only four hours of sleep.

Americans think it's *macho* to sleep in small amounts. Unfortunately, in this age little mistakes can be catastrophic . . . the wreck of a 747, an out of control nuclear reactor, a bus full of kids, or two trains on the same track going in different directions, for example.

Sleep deprivation hampers memory and mental alertness, disrupts vision and leaves you cranky and irritable all day long.

Adequate sleep is an essential ingredient to the joy of life.

When Do I Get The Most Restful Sleep?

Everyone's sleep patterns differ. However, according to some experts, the greatest depth of sleep is reached in the first two hours. This is followed by a less restful sleep and then one more deep sleep. Sleep quality is more important than sleep time. Complete relaxation is much more restorative than superficial, restless sleep. There are two types of sleepers. The evening type feels drowsy in the evening, falls asleep and is at his best in the morning. The morning sleeper is more fully alive in the evening. He falls asleep comparatively late, often with difficulty, and sleeps well into the late morning hours. If he has to get up earlier than he chooses, he feels bad and is disinclined to work.

Do People Wake Up Differently?

You can only wake up as fast as you warm up.

Efficiency in the morning has a direct connection with body temperature. Some people warm up faster, therefore wake up faster than others.

Nutritionists say that slow wakers may be deficient in protein and the B-complex vitamins.

The brain wakes you in a reverse order from which it put you to sleep. In a gradual progression, first your large muscles wake up — legs, arms, back and neck. Then come your senses. The first of these to wake is touch, then hearing, vision, and lastly smell.

Some people with a more vivid recollection of the cave days wake up at about four in the morning and have to have a bit of food before going back to sleep. This may be in recognition of the early rising of our ancestors when the night chill began to be erased by the early sun. The adrenal glands begin to do their job and the 4 o'clock riser is stirred into action. Since there's no fire to stoke and no reason to stay awake, a bite of cheese or a spoon of yogurt will quiet the adrenals and permit the person to go back to bed.

Will Sleeping Pills Help?

Consult a doctor. Sleeping pills interfere with rapid eye movement (REM) and prevent dreaming. That results in unproductive sleep and a stuffy-feeling morning. Many types of sleep medications lose their effect after two or three weeks of continual use. Regular use for more than a few nights running is not recommended. The only justifiable reason for their use is when there is an external trauma, such as a death in the family, when drugged sleep is better than grief.

Sleeping pills are not for pregnant women. They also tend to affect driving or operating machinery. It's best to consult a health professional to find out why you are not sleeping rather than resort to a possibly dangerous drug.

Which Is Best, A Hot Or A Cold Bedroom?

One in which you are most comfortable. Sleeping in a cold room used to be a must but that's an "old wives tale." Fresh air is a must, but temperature is an individual requirement. Researchers have discovered that low temperatures can influence dreams. Dreams can become more emotional and more unpleasant as the temperature in the room drops.

Does An Exercise Program Promote Good Sleep?

Regular exercise will help you sleep longer and better, but not if you exercise just before bedtime. A vigorous routine in the late evening will be stimulating and cause stress. Do your exercise routine in the early evening and get the sleep benefits later that night.

How About A Couple Or More Shots Of Alcohol . . .
How Will That Affect Sleep?

One glass of wine, a beer, or one ounce of alcohol can be relaxing and help tense people sleep better. More than one ounce can lead to fragmented and disturbed sleep. Chronic alcohol drinking will actually interfere with sleep. There is also the obvious danger of mixing alcohol and sleeping pills. The combination can depress the central nervous system to a dangerous extent, in some cases even causing death.

Sleepytime Herbs

The use of sleeping pills — prescription or over-the-counter — can be very dangerous to anyone suffering from sleep apnea. These drugs depress the respiratory system and can cause breathing to stop more often and for a longer period of time. Sleeping pills, alcohol, antihistamines and other central nervous system depressants may actually kill! Common sleeping pills — benzodiazepine and barbiturates — are depressing, says Dr. Andrew Weil, practicing physician and author of *Natural Health, Natural Medicine* (Houghton, Mifflin). They are addictive and dangerous if taken regularly.

But, what can you do if you need some kind of help to fall asleep?

Gentle, non-toxic herbs make the kind of tea you can drink safely at night and get the kind of refreshing sleep you want and need.

No prescription needed. Just walk into your health food store and pick up some herbal tea bags designed for sleep, with a combination of grandma-tested herbs, or get some single herbs and brew your own.

Grandma-tested is not quite fair since many herbs have been laboratory tested and just as well. One of the best is chamomile. Long recognized by traditional herbalism as a harmless sedative, chamomile was tested by Lawrence Gould, M.D., and colleagues who reported their findings in the Journal of *Clinical Pharmacology,* January 10, 1974. Actually, they weren't testing the herb for its benefits in inducing sleep. They wanted to find out if it had any ill effects on a group of cardiac patients who had undergone ventricular catheterization. As it turned out, chamomile had no cardiac effects but there was a positive reaction of another kind.

The medical team reported that "a striking sleep-inducing action of the tea was noted in 10 of 12 patients. It is most unusual for patients undergoing cardiac catheterizations to fall asleep. The anxiety produced by this procedure, as well as the pain associated with cardiac catheterization, all but precludes sleep. Thus, the fact that 10 of 12 patients fell into a deep slumber after drinking chamomile tea is all the more striking."

Wow! It would appear that if someone can fall asleep right after undergoing a painful medical procedure, your problem should disappear after two gulps.

Either buy the tea bags or collect a handful of the flowers, pour a cup of boiling water over them and let them steep for ten minutes. Then strain, add honey to taste and goodnight!

Many other herbs can also solve your sleep problems. Here's a sampler of the best. Since we are all individuals, what works best for one may not work for all. Try them until you find a couple that work well for you.

Aromatic Woodruff

Here's a nice mixture that combines wine and this herb. Make a cup of tea with the herb, using hot, not boiling, water. Warm up one ounce of a good wine and add it to the cup. Sprinkle some cinnamon, add a bit of honey and stir. Sip away until you begin to nod *and then go to bed.*

Catnip

You don't have to fight your cat for his favorite catnip mouse. Catnip herb is available in health food stores and tea bags are also on hand. The same chemicals in catnip that drive your kitty into a drunken frenzy are sedatives to you. It's safe and non-toxic with a minty taste.

Hops

You've tasted hops if you've ever had a glass of beer. But tea made with hops is one of the best sleep-inducers you can find. The sedative chemical in hops was isolated by a science team in 1983. So the old wives tale that hops makes you sleepy was found to be true. Take a couple of teaspoons of hops and put them in a cup. Add boiling water and let steep for five minutes. Strain, add honey to taste and that's that.

Passionflower

Won't arouse your passion despite its name, but it can soothe your nerves and help you sleep. Passionflower contains a combination which gives a tea made from this flower a mild sedative/tranquilizing effect. Alone or as part of a sleeping potion, passionflower is a well-regarded European herb. Some people react to one of the ingredients with mild stomach upset. If that happens, use a different herb. No use trading in one complaint for another.

Balm

Balm is considered another of nature's natural tranquilizers. Its use is well documented, especially in Germany where it is prescribed as a sedative/tranquilizer when the stronger, pharmaceutical products are not necessary. You may have to take two cups of tea to get its sleep-producing effect.

Skullcap

Strange name for a herb but that doesn't take away from its ability to calm frazzled nerves. One drawback is its bitter taste so use honey to sweeten it enough for you to profit from its sedative use. Russians swear by its ability, as does much of the European community.

Steep it for ten to fifteen minutes in order to extract all of its power.

Sage

Sage tea with a little honey can make you very comfortable. Mix one teaspoonful of sage, one teaspoonful of rosemary and two teaspoonfuls of peppermint leaves together. Use one teaspoonful of the mixture to a cup of boiling water. Steep for five minutes, strain, add honey to taste and get to bed.

Lemon Balm

This herb tea will not "put" you to sleep the way some other herbs will. Lemon balm tends to relax you and take away some of the strain and tension that stands between you and a good night's rest. It also doubles as an early morning tea to help take away spasms and help overcome a feeling of tiredness.

Wild Cherry

Although usually thought of as a cough or cold remedy, Wild Cherry can be very helpful for incomnia. It acts as a sedative and tranquilizing agent. You'll find it useful for anxiety and stress as well as sleeplessness. However, don't have more than three cups a day. Hydrocyanic acid, its main chemical ingredient, is a relative of cyanide, the poison, so follow directions carefully. You want a good night's sleep. . .not The Big Sleep!

Yarrow

The American Indians used this herb for a number of ailments, particularly arthritis. It contains a hypnotic chemical called thujone. Take two teaspoons of yarrow to a cup of boiling water and let it steep for ten to fifteen minutes. Strain, add honey to taste and sip.

Valerian

This herb is frequently used as part of an herbal sleep formula, either in a capsule or in a tablet. It's wonderful for sleep (its ingredients served as the basis for the formulation of VALIUM). However, it's not habit forming or harmful unless you consider its odor.

Valerian smells, to put it kindly, like an old sock. But, if you can ignore its odor and drink the tea, you'll sleep like a baby. It has the added value of being able to lower your blood pressure at the same time. Valerian has a long history in this country and has been used since Colonial times.

Health food stores also sell herbal sleeping potions in capsule or tablet form.

A typical formula will include these herbs:

- Valerian
- Hops
- Skullcap
- Passionflower

The usual dose is 2 capsules twenty minutes before bedtime.

They can be effective in helping to promote a restful night's sleep. However, like any other artificial means of combatting insomnia, they will not ease the underlying cause. If insomnia lasts for a period of weeks, seek the help of a health professional.

A SECOND LAST-MINUTE GIFT

Gamma-Oryzanol — The Anti-Pot-Belly Pill

It's a shame but most people, as they age, tend to lose muscle tissue and assume that pot-bellied stance we associate with the elderly. One of the reasons is a lack of exercise and another is the reluctance of the body to build muscle instead of fat.

Gamma-oryzanol is a new energy aid that can increase body mass, decrease fatty tissue and help fight the free radicals that invade your body, causing cellular destruction and making the body look old and sagging.

Gamma-oryzanol was discovered more than thirty years ago when it was extracted from rice bran by Japanese scientists. Even though it is thirty years old, it has only recently come to the attention of the public. It began with bodybuilders who wanted to get more from their workouts. They discovered that GO influences the hypothalamus in the brain which in turn governs the pituitary gland and through it a number of the body's automatic functions including hormonal regulation.

Those hormones include the sex hormones (testosterone in the male and estrogen in the female. These hormones help to build muscles and to develop a better appearance.

Another important benefit is that it appears to relieve many of the annoying symptoms of menopause-related problems. It also acts as an antioxidant helping to neutralize chemical particles known as free radicals from both outside of the body and from inside the body. Vitamin E and selenium are two nutrients which help control free radicals and GO is a new member of the protective team.

GO is available from health food stores and drugstores and should be used according to label instructions. If you use it with Vitamin E then combine 20 mg of GO with 100 I.U. of vitamin E.

Now let's instantly correct the fatal error that almost everyone makes when they do situps. Unless you correct this, you're actually shaping your stomach into a round ball, instead of the slim, flat, hard, tucked-in "gut of steel" you want.

When you lay down, cross your hands on your stomach, and not behind your back. Bend your knees, so they're raised. Then, *before* you come up, exhale through your mouth, until every drop of air is forced out of your stomach.

As the air is forced out, pull in your gut. When you come up, that gut should be empty and flat.

Now, come up about six inches, and count to a lucky seven. Then lower your upper torso again. Then, repeat for as many sets of ten as you feel comfortable with. Rest one minute between each group, of course.

INDEX

B

C